THROUGH THE BARREN TREES

Merry -
With gratitude
for your friendship -
Great is God's
faithfulness!
Karey Kline
3-19-02

Booklocker.com, Inc.
2001

Through the Barren Trees

Nancy Kline

For Jeremy and Zachary, the best chips
Richard Kline ever made

Table of Contents

Acknowledgments

When I started this book, I thought that it would be time consuming but fulfilling. I also assumed that I could do it on my own. I was wrong. I could never have completed this manuscript without the consistent and loving encouragement of friends and family members.

Equally valuable was the technical support of friends who read my very unpolished work and individually gave me suggestions to transform my rambling memories to a cohesive piece of writing. Thanks to Arlene Teich and Barb Ludwig who read the beginnings of my very first draft and encouraged me to give it more "structure". I am very grateful for Steve Miller's painstaking review of the first fifty pages and his line by line suggestions to make the stories and ideas more cohesive.

When I thought the book was "done", my brother Ray and sister-in-law Jan helped me to see that it could still be "cleaned up". Their insights were invaluable.

Finally, many thanks to my coworker Helene Brady who willingly took on the tedious task of final editing.

Preface

When cancer strikes, it does not do its damage in some isolated laboratory; it affects living human beings and those they love. It struck our family when my husband Dick was diagnosed with colorectal cancer in February, 1998. This is a story about cancer, but it is also a chronicle of our family's life together and our faith in God throughout the years of Dick's illness.

Part of the story is in Dick's own words, in the form of emails that he wrote to friends and relatives. While I have included some of my emails as well, most of my writing is taken from the journal which I began shortly after Dick first became ill. The emails are more plentiful in the latter part of the book, as Dick chose to share more of his experience.

We had the privilege of sharing our story with many friends as it unfolded. We received countless affirmations of how our faith positively impacted those who witnessed it. May this narrative of our journey be an encouragement to you as well.

Lightening Strikes:

August 12, 2000; March 1998

Chapter 1

August 12, 2000

"Nance, please help me die." That was Dick's request when I stopped by his bed earlier today to see if he needed anything.

I know that these words were not a plea for assisted suicide; he was just indicating a readiness to go. Until a few days ago, morphine had been effective in controlling his head and neck pain, but new pain from bladder spasms has made him uncomfortable again.

"Okay, Hon," I tearfully answered. "I'll do what I can. I'll keep giving you the pain medication - as much as you need to stay comfortable. You can go."

I know that I need to let him go, and I long for him to be done with pain and suffering, but I can't imagine his not being here any more.

****

January 2001

Dick and I had been together for about half of our lives when he was first diagnosed with cancer in February 1998. We met in 1973, having both just graduated from college. Dick came east from his home and college in Syracuse, New York, to attend graduate school for electrical engineering at MIT (Massachusetts Institute of Technology), just a few months after I moved to Boston for my first nursing job.

We met in Cambridge at a Bible study group. The group convened in the home of eight or nine young adults who shared a faith in God and lived together in "Christian community". Though Dick and I liked each other, at first there was no attraction beyond a basic friendship. Dick was briefly engaged to be married when we first met, and he was just "not my type". He was a poor, studious graduate student, and I was gainfully employed and ready to party. Nonetheless, in the fall of 1974, when several people moved out of the community, my roommate Beth and I moved in at the same time that Dick did.

Starting at that point, the friendship between Dick and me began to blossom into love, and we married in 1976. A year later, Dick finished his time at MIT - just a thesis short of his PhD. He had decided that being a full-time student was not compatible with marriage, and he felt that our marriage was more important than schooling. I often felt guilty about his decision to end his formal education. I knew that he aspired to teach at the university level, and he needed a PhD to be a professor. After many years, I finally accepted that the decision Dick made was not so much a sacrifice as a well thought out choice, a choice that indicated how highly he valued our marriage.

Our first child, Jeremy, was born in 1979, and despite the fact that he had complications at birth, he had no residual deficits, and clearly inherited his father's math genius and his mother's outgoing personality. Zachary, born 3 years later, inherited his father's analytic mind as well as his gentle spirit. As the boys grew, other similarities to their parents became apparent. Jeremy and I tend to make it well known how we are feeling - you might call us "high maintenance people" - while Zach and Dick shared a tendency to reservedness: both preferring to keep their thoughts to themselves.

Over the years it became apparent that certain things were important to our family: God, laughter and time together. We laughed a lot: at our daily suppers together; our Sunday breakfasts and lunches together; and on our many vacations together. As the boys grew older, we abandoned the Sunday afternoon outings that we used to take, and our weekend trips became much less frequent, but I attempted to plan at least one good family vacation a year. We had some fine vacations trips both bc and ac (before and after children): touring the national parks of the southwest; exploring Nova Scotia; enjoying the rides and activities of Disney World in Florida; walking the beaches on Cape Cod here in Massachusetts; touring the Midwest while visiting friends; vacationing at Christian family camps; visiting my brother Ray and his family in Tanzania and Kenya; whitewater rafting in Maine and western Massachusetts; and backpacking in the White Mountains of New Hampshire.

We had planned to go to Haiti for a missions trip in April, 1998 - a last big vacation before Jeremy graduated from high school - but we heard of some violent attacks on tourists there, and we questioned if it was wise to put our lives in danger. We chose instead to give a donation to the mission we had intended to visit, and we planned a trip to Cancun - to relax and enjoy the sun south of the border.

We had been very fortunate to enjoy good health in our family of four. Other than Jeremy's birth problems and a back problem for Dick, we were essentially strangers to illness prior to Dick's diagnosis of cancer. We got the news as I was preparing to leave on a church youth retreat with Zach and Jeremy and about 30 other teenagers. Since just before Jeremy started high school, I had been working as a volunteer youth leader for our church, and going on retreats was something that I had always enjoyed. This was the first retreat for which both Jeremy and Zachary were of the appropriate age to go, so Dick was home alone for the weekend.

The beginning of our experience with cancer is probably best described in Dick's words, in an email he sent to my brother and sister-in-law, Ray and Jan. They had been living in Africa for about thirteen years, working as physicians for missions organizations. We had been able to communicate with them much more easily and frequently since they gained access to a computer and internet capabilities. This is the email that Dick wrote to Ray and Jan while Jeremy, Zach and I were away.

****

March 1, 1998

I was doing some reading this weekend and came across the following information that you might be interested in (recent medical research which I stumbled across on the web). "Cancer of the colon is a highly treatable and often curable disease when localized to the bowel. It is the second most frequent cause of cancer death. Surgery is the primary treatment and results in cure in approximately 50% of the patients. Recurrence following surgery is a major problem and often is the ultimate cause of death." Now in the past, such trivial information would have been of little interest to me. Previously most of my reading was centered around object oriented programming and how one can use polymorphism (a fancy name for virtual functions) to define and implement class hierarchies such that you can define base class behavior and methods which will manipulate future instances (a fancy name for objects) of a yet to be conceived classes. However, it seems, now that I have been diagnosed with colon cancer, that all of a sudden I have developed a taste for other interesting bathroom reading material when sitting on the can.

I have to admit that I was a bit taken aback when I read that first part about "results in cure in approximately 50% of the patients". Immediately what came to my mind (being an astute engineer, well-equipped in mathematics) was, "Wait a minute, what happens to the other 50%? You doctors, why can't you just call a spade, a spade and come right out and say it, 'We try, but we really can't help everyone.

4

Those other 50%, well, it's hard to put in writing, but they...'" Oh well, you get the idea.

Although I was "taken aback" at first when I read the above, I then turned and looked at it from a Biblical perspective. God knows the number of hairs on my head (that alone is quite a task, given that the number decreases every day) and He knew me even before I was in the womb. He knew the day and hour that I was going to be born, and He knows the day and the hour when He is going to call me home, be it in a few hours, or in another 50 years from now. As I told my pastor, I know with God, it's not just one big crap shoot (oops, a bad word!)

Well, now, let's get serious; enough with this joking around. Let me give you a brief history of the events of the past couple of months, and especially, the past couple of days, so that you can be praying for us. I started to pass blood (a lot of blood) in my stool sometime in early January. The first thought that entered my mind is that this is not good for a 47-year old male. After about two or three days of the same, I called my doctor. I came into the office, he did the normal stick the finger up the butt, said it was probably hemorrhoids and told me to take hot baths and to stick these medicated suppositories up my butt. (Sorry if I don't have all the right medical lingo, but you probably can translate for me.) He also said, since you are almost 50, I am going to schedule you for a flexible sigmoid blah, blah, blah... with a specialist. Had to wait about 30 days for that appointment. This guy (who luckily had a very nice bedside manner - important in the medical profession, if you ask me) stuck an 18" flexible tube up my butt. Now according to the same article that I quoted from earlier, supposedly, this doesn't cause the patient much discomfort, usually resulting in a slight sensation of pressure. Well, let me tell you, I'd like to get the researcher who wrote that article on the table and let me stick that thing up his butt; it hurts like *&^%&^(*!

After that exam, the doctor said he had good news, and bad news. The good news was that my colon looked great. The bad news was, my colon looked great, so why am I bleeding? So, he wrote me a prescription for some medicated suppositories, and told be to call him back in a couple of weeks if the bleeding didn't stop. Well, I called back in a couple of weeks when the bleeding didn't stop and he scheduled me for a complete colonoscopy. You know, that's when they a stick a 6 foot flexible tube up your butt; but luckily, I was asleep for this, so I didn't feel a thing.

This happened last Thursday. They found and biopsied the tumor. It turns out that it is very close to my rectum (they don't know why they didn't see it with the 18" version, since it is only 6" or 8" in - probably because I was feeling a mild sensation of pressure!). On Friday the pathology report came back that it is cancer. Friday afternoon after receiving the report, I spent the afternoon on the phone arranging visits and further tests for this week. Thursday is probably the day we will learn the most: CAT scan in the morning, which will give further information on the size and extent of the tumor, and then Thursday afternoon we meet with the surgeon who will be doing the operation. I'm writing this note so that you'll pray with us. Please pray for:
- Thursday, that the CAT scan may show the tumor to be small and localized.
- Operation, hopefully sometime soon (next week).
- That the nasty cold and cough that I have now will go away soon and not delay the operation.
- For God's grace and peace.
Thanks,
Dick

****

March 1, 1998
I didn't see this email to Ray and Jan until I got back today from the youth retreat. Dick sounds so calm in his writing. I guess I am, too, even though it all seems so unreal. Before I left two days ago, I talked to Dick from the church office as we were preparing to leave, and he insisted there was no reason for me not to go. He also gave me permission to tell other people about the cancer. This was important for me, but uncharacteristic for him, since he is usually so private. He said it was okay because "the more people that are praying, the better." I told the boys first, before we left. Having had no experience with cancer before, they were saddened, but confident that the doctors would take care of the problem and that their dad would be fine.

While driving to New Hampshire, I told my good friend Carolyn, another of the youth leaders, and the next day when the rest of the leaders were relaxing together after breakfast, Carolyn and I told them all. We prayed together. For us as adults, the word cancer generates more fear than it does for those who are younger and have not seen its devastating effects. I appreciated those adults, who were all very supportive of me.

Later in the day, I had two experiences that were both encouraging and a bit disturbing. Twice I took long walks with other people. In both cases I was really the "odd" person – an unintended addition to a couple - but in each situation I had the feeling that it was OKAY. I enjoyed myself, and did not feel like a fifth wheel. I found that comforting, but at the same time unsettling. I hope Dick's having cancer doesn't mean that I will someday be alone. I feel ridiculous even entertaining that thought. I expect he'll just have the surgery and he'll be fine.

I also feel ridiculous that even though I'm a nurse, it never occurred to me that Dick might have cancer. His bleeding had been bright red – "frank" bleeding as opposed to "occult" bleeding (hidden in the stool from higher up in the digestive tract) so I just thought it was a bleeding polyp or some irritation along the lower intestinal wall. I guess it doesn't really matter now what I thought. Even though he had been bleeding since the beginning of January – two months ago – I guess cancers are often around for quite a while before they make themselves known by obvious symptoms, so my considering the possibility of cancer last month really wouldn't have made any difference in the long run.

I don't feel particularly sad. I'm acutely aware - and have been for some time - that Dick and I are incredibly blessed. Despite this knowledge, I have had moments when I thought that because everything was going so well, something terrible was going to happen - like Dick dying in a plane crash or something. I finally gave up thinking those negative thoughts and decided instead to focus on being thankful. Even now, I don't feel that the cancer is "the bad thing" that I feared, but rather that, like Job, we need to accept the bad as well as the good. The rain falls and the sun rises and sets on the just and the unjust alike.

Even though I don't feel particularly sad, I did have some tearful moments during the weekend at the retreat. Most of them came when we were singing worship songs, like "You are my strength when I am weak; You are the treasure that I seek; You are my all in all." It was overwhelming to think of my weakness when facing something as powerful as cancer, but my tears were also tears of joy that I do have a Source of strength when I can't deal with life's struggles on my own. I called Dick from the retreat, and he told me that he, too, had shed tears. He felt it was good for him to be alone to begin to process "the news" of the cancer.

THROUGH THE BARREN TREES

I'm glad I went on the retreat, but it sure is good to be back home again with Dick.

Chapter 2

March 7, 1998
Another email from Dick, sent while my sister Mary Ellen and brother-in-law Phil were visiting Ray and Jan in Kenya

Just another letter from your jealous and envious brother-in-law who is stuck here in the states while his other "relations" are gallivanting about the beautiful scenery, peoples, and culture of Eastern Africa. Please pay no attention to my cynicism.

Thank you for your note, and for your prayers. First, an update on your prayers, which to date appear to have been answered, but please keep praying about the situation for the next four or five years.

Had my blood tests Monday and the CAT scan Thursday. The first good news came Wednesday evening. God knows when we need a pick-me-up because I (we?) had been doing pretty good up to that point, but were just starting to get a little bit anxious and I'm afraid, starting to fear the worst. As you may know, this seems to happen sometimes when you're waiting for something to happen and you go through a period of no news. Well, this appeared to be the case by Wednesday night as we were waiting for Thursday to arrive all week (i.e., CAT scan, and meet the surgeon). Well, Wednesday evening my primary physician called about 8:00 P.M. to inform us that my blood tests had come back and the news was all good. The blood tests showed two things: first of all that my liver is functioning normally, and second, that my CEA(?) level was low. Apparently, if the cancer had started to spread to elsewhere in my body (stage 4?), then there would be a high probability that my CEA level would have been high. It wasn't much news, but it was all good news, and it was just what we needed at the time to pick our spirits up for Thursday (God is good).

I had the CAT scan Thursday morning at Faulkner hospital. Had to go in early (7:00). Had to drink about 20 ounces of some chemical that they covered up with strawberry esters [flavor]. Had my second IV of the week (the first of many I'm sure – hard for a guy who faints when he sees needles, or when his in-laws start talking about the high cholesterol levels in the shellfish that he is presently eating). But I have to say that God's grace was there through it all and that I really felt God's peace. (It helped that I was still flying high from the good news of Wednesday evening).

Nancy and I met with the surgeon late Thursday afternoon. Mostly good news. He looked at the CAT scan. I thought he would study it intently, but to my surprise he just threw it up on the lighted thing on the wall and quickly glanced at each of the sixty or so images. I had also thought (hoped) that he would have seen the tumor in the images, but he explained that the colon doesn't image all that well and the main reason for the CAT scan was to look at the liver, and the good news is that my liver looks normal.

He stuck that "thing" up my butt to get a first hand look at the tumor himself. The biggest concern is the location of the tumor. It appears to be about 9 cm from the rectum. A few more, and the operation would be relatively straightforward. A few less and they probably would not be able to save the rectum. He can't say for certain what the outcome will be until they actually do the operation, but the most likely scenario that he can paint at the present time is that he will be able to save the rectum (depending upon if the tumor has "invaded the fatty tissues" or not) and that I will end up with a temporary ileostomy for about eight weeks, allowing for the colon / rectum resection to completely heal before pressing it back into service "doing its job".

Post op adjunct therapy depends upon the stage of the cancer, which he won't know for sure until a few days after the operation. If I'm a stage II or III, then radiation and chemo will be used. If I'm a stage I, then there doesn't appear to be any advantage to radiation or chemo. His best guess is that I'm either stage I or II.

Surgery is scheduled for Tuesday. Monday I have four different appointments at three different locations ranging from Norwood to Boston (the curse of the modern automobile and HMO's) [Health Maintenance Organizations]. *Weather report for Monday is not good (rain, 60 mile per hour winds!).*

Please continue to pray for God's grace and peace, as I know you will.

Thanks,
Dick

****

March 7, 1998
I went with Dick for the appointment with the surgeon, Dr. Bleday. He seems a pleasant fellow. He essentially ignored me when we first met, but I think that was because he wanted to be sure to focus on Dick.

He's the same doctor who operated on a teacher who works at the school where I am the school nurse. Kim has the same kind of cancer as Dick, and after her surgery, Dr. Bleday reportedly told her brother, "You'll be lucky if your sister is alive in three years." So, I guess he's pretty blunt, and if he says anything positive to us, we figure that we can feel really good about it!

When Dr. Bleday explained the surgery to us, in addition to mentioning the possibility of an ileostomy (pulling the small intestines out through the abdomen, so Dick would have to wear a bag to collect his stool), he told us that impotence or sterility is a problem in about 25% of these kinds of surgeries. Sterility is not an issue for us, since we don't want more children at this stage of our lives anyway, but the thought of either impotence or an ileostomy doesn't thrill Dick or me. I guess I idealistically thought that we could just get rid of the cancer and not have to worry about anything <u>bad</u> coming from the procedure that is supposed to be life-giving. I really don't want our life as we now know it to be altered at all. I'd be quite content for things to return to exactly the way they were before we heard about the cancer!

Although we know that we must face the possibility of complications, we understand that Dr. Bleday specializes in nerve sparing surgery, so at least we have a good shot at getting the job done the best that it can be.

****

March 9, 1998

One of Dick's pre-op appointments today was in Dr. Bleday's office with an ostomy nurse. They needed to "mark" him in case he needs an ileostomy. The doctor and nurse like to see the patient prior to the surgery, wearing regular clothes, so that they don't end up putting the stoma (the end of the intestines that comes out through the skin) in a place where it would be irritated by his pant's waistline or belt. Dick expected that they might use a permanent marker to note the location for the stoma, but instead the nurse actually <u>cut</u> him, scratching an inch long X on his belly with a needle. I was quite surprised by that - wondered if it was really necessary...

****

11

March 10, 1998 - Surgery Day

I always had thought if someone close to me had surgery, I'd be at the hospital waiting nearby, and then the surgeon would come out, like they do on television, and tell me that "the surgery went well, and you'll be able to see him soon." Well, I guess reality is always a little different than TV; Dr. Bleday had convinced me that there was no need for me to be at the hospital during the surgery. Besides, the surgery was scheduled for noon and was expected to take three hours, so I wouldn't be able to see Dick anyway until after work was over for me. So, I went to work, thankful to be busy instead of just waiting alone by the phone. I made sure Dr. Bleday had both my work and home numbers, and I knew that the boys would be home before me, so they could answer the phone if the doctor should call while I was en route from work.

He called just after I arrived home, at 3:30, telling me first that "it was a difficult intubation" because Dick's larynx sits farther forward in his neck than most, and he expected that Dick would not have pleasant memories of the intubation experience. When I asked about the cancer, he said that it appears that they got it all, and he got a good margin around the tumor. It doesn't appear that there was any cancer in the surrounding tissue or in the lymph nodes, but we won't know for sure until the pathologist's report comes back on Friday. He didn't need to do an ileostomy!

The boys and I got to the hospital around 6:45, expecting that Dick would be in his room, but it turned out to be a one and a half hour wait. We passed the time playing volleyball in the waiting area with a squashed Styrofoam cup; spinning coins on the floor by the elevator; and watching a little TV in his room-to-be. We're fairly good at entertaining ourselves, but it was a bit tedious waiting for so long. When Dick finally did come up from the recovery room, we were amazed at how alert he was and how good he looked. We all feel there is reason to be hopeful.

****

March 13, 1998
Email from me to Ray and Jan
Title: "Not So Up Update"

Please don't let up on the prayers for Dick. It's stage III. Not the news we expected or hoped for. It hadn't looked like the cancer had spread through the bowel wall, but it had. 2 of the 5 lymph nodes were positive. Of course they are gone now, but as we all know, those nasty little cancer cells can be hiding, so Dick will need adjuvant therapies, as they say, to raise his "cure" chances from 40% to 60%. (Why am I not thrilled at those numbers?)

The surgeon came in as I was leaving the hospital tonight around 9:15. We'll have to see the oncologist and radiologist, but the surgeon indicated that those therapies should begin within 6 weeks, so we'll prob go to Cancun as planned, then he'll start six weeks of daily radiation with a continuous pump of chemo (leuko-something, I think) and some 5FU, too.

I'm feeling sad now. Up to now, the news was all either unknown or good, and this last bit's a bit tough to swallow. (Nobody is up for me to call at 11:45PM, so you lucky guys get to be my sounding board.) I know for certain that God is in control and that he loves us very much, and there is no question that we are very blessed, and I know I have no more reason to ask "why this?" than to ask why we are so blessed, but all that knowledge doesn't make me any less sad as I try to grasp the reality of this. Can't we just go back to before this all started? But that wouldn't help, because the doctor said this cancer has probably been there for 4-5 years, and there have been many wonderful things in our lives in the past 5 years.

Okay. For the looking on the bright side - if we didn't have the possibility of the microscopic studies, we wouldn't know that the cancer was in the lymph nodes, and we wouldn't be doing the radiation and the chemo to kill off those invisible little buggers (albeit, while killing off some good stuff down there, too. But no, this was supposed to be the "bright side" paragraph.) Okay, for the other good news, Dick is healing remarkably well and will probably come home tomorrow ('cause the insurance company thinks it's time for him to go.) Actually, the doctor thinks it's fine for him to come home as long as he feels okay when he eats. (He's had no solid foods yet, but is passing gas quite nicely.) He's been walking around a lot, and the pain seems under control without excessive medication. He looks great!

I'm tired. I don't relish the thought of telling everyone whom I've just told that things look great that things aren't all that great. But then again, God is Great and God is good (and we thank Him...) Thanks for listening and bearing this burden with me. I'm going to try to work on a more upbeat presentation now that I've got that all out.

Love,
Nance

****

March 13, 1998

I've been able to handle everything (the cancer and the surgery) reasonably well up to now, but this news of the cancer not being confined has put me over the edge. I cried on Dick's shoulder in the hospital tonight, but it was hard to get a really good hug because of the discomfort of his incision. I cried because the news is unexpected; I really thought the cancer was all gone. I cried for the future of discomfort that Dick now faces with the radiation and chemo, and I cried for potential losses. Does this mean a shorter life expectancy for Dick? Will radiation damage him permanently – maybe make him impotent? If the cancer comes back, will that mean a colostomy for Dick?

I cried for a long time, but I couldn't stay at the hospital all night, so I dried my tears and went out to the parking lot. It was rather late when I left – actually late enough that I didn't have to pay to leave the parking lot – a nice little plus in the middle of some big minuses! I knew that I would have a half hour drive home, so I took a lot of deep breaths in an effort to keep from crying again. I flipped on the car radio to distract myself, but soon shut it off again because I found it so annoying.

I arrived safely home and told Zach the sad news about the cancer not being confined. Again I cried.

****

March 14, 1998

I woke up this morning ready to be done with crying, but that's not so easy. After the boys left to go out to breakfast, I got up after crying just a bit, and the phone rang. It was Nadjia. She's someone from church who has very rarely called here. She wanted to know where to mail a get well card for Dick. She asked how Dick was doing, and I told her the news: that the cancer is in the lymph nodes, and he needs chemotherapy and radiation. I tried to be matter-of-fact as I told her, but those darn tears started up again. Of all the people I know, there could have been no better person to talk to at that point than Nadjia. She's been in my shoes - only her situation was a lot tougher. When her husband was diagnosed with cancer and died many years ago, her boys were very young. She understood why I was crying, and she understood when I told her that I know for sure that God is in control, but right now I feel so very out of control. She assured me that God's being in control

14

and my being in control are two completely different things. He is <u>still</u> in control even when I feel helpless. After our conversation, I felt remarkably refreshed and strengthened, with a sense that God's timing - for this particular phone call - was quite remarkable.

During my conversation with Nadjia, the boys were out for breakfast. Saturday breakfast out is the usual Saturday morning routine, but this is the first time ever that they had gone without Dad. They've had this Saturday breakfast tradition ever since Zach was a toddler and just couldn't handle going out for supper (he'd literally climb the walls in the restaurant!) but seemed more able to deal with a restaurant earlier in the day. Anyway, Dick started taking the boys out while I slept in. As they got older and I didn't need the break any more, it had become such a positive experience for the three of them that it has continued right through the high school years.

It is amazing to me that the mundane – and not so mundane – things of life continue, even when cancer is now part of our life. One of these things - the smashed windshield - we had hoped to address before Dick got home, but since he's coming home today, I guess he'll have to find out about it. It happened Wednesday or Thursday. Turns out it was all because of a high school French project. The assignment was for the students to make a video using some vocabulary words they had been learning related to *les voitures* (automobiles). Jeremy and his friends planned to show in a video the kinds of things that one should <u>avoid</u> doing with automobiles, such as standing near a puddle when a car drives by, or drinking and driving, or standing in <u>front</u> of a moving vehicle. It was this last that led to the ultimate demise of the windshield. Apparently the boys decided that an authentic looking video of a car hitting a person would necessitate said person (Pete, in this case) jumping on the hood of the car when "hit". Now Pete, to be quite dramatic, reportedly made a flying leap, unwittingly bypassing the hood and landing – elbow first – on the windshield of Jeremy's 1989 Taurus station wagon. Pete wasn't hurt, but the windshield was thoroughly cracked. To his credit, Jeremy did some investigating and negotiating and managed to get a rock bottom price for the windshield replacement.

Sometimes even problems can be a welcome diversion from the constant focus on cancer.

Mostly Cloudy:

March 1998 - April 1998

Chapter 3

March 22.1998
Email from me to Ray and Jan

The latest update is that we now have a plan for further treatment. We saw an oncologist last Tuesday (the one to which Dick's primary care (internist) physician referred us), and we weren't impressed. Comments like "Yours is a pretty serious case," and "I haven't ever used this particular protocol for cancer treatment, but I'll read up on it," did not inspire confidence. Now if I were in Africa, and I needed surgery, I'd be happy to go to either of you, but if I lived here and had a choice between you or somebody who had done the kind of surgery that I needed a zillion times, I'd go for the zillion timer. Likewise, we decided that since we are near Boston and a fair amount of cancer experience, we'd look a bit further for an experienced oncologist. We saw him on Thursday - the doctor that Dick's surgeon had suggested and who was mentioned by other folks as well - particularly experienced in this field of cancer. We also have an appointment this week with a radiologist who has had a lot of experience of shooting the rays in this area of the belly.

The plan is to be in a clinical trial - Dick will be randomly selected for one of three groups - one of them being conventional treatment, and the other 2 being slight variations on that. The protocol calls for treatment to begin 20-70 days post surgery, so we still plan to go to Cancun. (We no longer wonder why it didn't work out to do a missions trip then, but as Dick points out, we probably wouldn't have appreciated it last November if God had said, "You can't go to Haiti in April because Dick has cancer.") The docs feel this will be a good rest, and Dick has an appointment the Monday after we return to get blood work done and begin the chemo. The plan is for 2 months of chemo (either continuous infusion or via injection - 5 days then 3 weeks rest, then 5 days and 3 weeks rest); then 6 weeks radiation (daily) plus chemo; then 4 weeks rest; then 2 more months chemo like the first round. It sounds like a long haul, but at least it will be during good weather, and I'll be off work for a couple of months of the treatment. One day at a time.

Jeremy got into Webb Institute - that little (90 students) free (non-military) school for Naval Architecture and Marine Engineering on Long Island. He liked it a lot when he visited it, but he's going to University of

17

Virginia next weekend to check that out again, and then revisit Webb for a close comparison.
    Lots happening here!
    One day at a time.
     Love,
     Nance

****

    I can't believe Jeremy is really getting ready to decide about college. This Webb Institute sounds great to me, even though I haven't visited it. How can he go wrong with it? It's very competitive, yet he got in. There is a really great professor to student ratio, and Jeremy felt very confident and comfortable when he visited it. Nevertheless, I have to remember that it is his decision, not mine.

    There are so many important things that are out of my control right now: Dick's health, Jeremy's future, my future. I know that there is not much I can do to influence Dick's health and therefore my future, so I guess I want to grasp the illusion of control by trying to influence Jeremy's choice of college. I know that is not wise, but I do have trouble keeping my mouth shut!

    Dick, on the other hand, has always had a better sense of when to be quiet and when to speak. He asked to speak at our church this morning. This is a transcript of what he said:

    First of all, I would like to thank everyone for all your prayers and for all the cards I have received. It's hard to hold them in one's hand; there are so many cards. I thank you not because we are supporting Hallmark, but rather because of the messages that were contained within them: in particular the phrase that you were praying for me. I wanted you to know that those prayers were felt and they are certainly what got me through the past several weeks. As I told several people this morning, I'm probably not as well as I look, and yet, over the past couple of weeks, the healing from the surgery has been quite miraculous. I thank you.

    I ask that you would continue to pray for me. There is a road to go yet. During the next month I need to regain my strength and recover from the surgery. Starting at the end of April I'll begin about six months of chemo and radiation. It's hard to think of going through that, but I know I have your prayers supporting me. The surgeon has told me that even after that road that the probability of surviving five years or longer is only sixty percent, but I know that we don't deal in probabilities; God knows exactly what He is doing. I am completely within His love. Things are going to work out fine.

I want to share a word of testimony, but before that, I have to explain a little bit about myself. It's kind of hard, because the Scripture says we should do things in the closet, just between ourselves and God. But before I can explain about my testimony, I have to explain a little bit about myself.

I have been a Christian for 27 years and I think if you were to talk to people who have known me over that period of time - ask my family - they know I'm not perfect. I sin every day; I have a temper and I procrastinate; I'm too concerned about finances at times. There are certainly many failings, and yet if you were to talk to them, I think they would say, "Dick has a consistent direction in his life. He wants to praise God with his life."

I can give some simple examples of that. I recall when I had been a Christian for just a couple of years and the first job I got was as a teaching assistant at MIT. It only paid $400 a month, and it was not easy even back then to live in Boston on $400 a month. But I had been in God's Word, and it talked about tithing; it said you should give 10% to God, so when I got that check, I would set $40 aside. God has blessed; He says He will increase it 30, 60, or 100 fold. I've seen Him increase what we are able to give 40 fold in the years since.

Another example is when Nancy and I were married, we were somewhat surprised, but we admitted to each other about 6 months after our wedding that we were still both attracted to people of the opposite sex. But God's Word said to "be content with the wife of thy youth." We admitted our feelings to each other, and continued to love each other and chose to love each other and to reject anything else. I can tell you that God has blessed our marriage, and we have had almost 22 years now of a passionate love affair that has only increased each year during the 22 years that God has blessed us.

When I graduated from MIT, I had been studying all sorts of higher mathematics and engineering, and I didn't really realize it when I was studying it, but it was only really used for two things: one was to send man to the moon, and we had already done that and weren't doing it any more, and the other was to guide nuclear missiles to support what was referred to at the time as "mutually assured destruction." At that time, I had been reading the Sermon on the Mount which said, "Blessed are the Peacemakers". I knew that I could not take a job that was planning on the mass murder of millions of people. It was difficult at the time when I just got rejection letter after rejection letter telling me I was overqualified and a few letters saying, "Please, come interview with us," but they were from places like NSA and Los Alamos. Yet God has been faithful to more than supply for my needs over the years.

I share this with you not to say that I am perfect by any means, but over that 27 years there has been a persistent direction in my life: to glorify God, and when I say that it is so important, I encourage you to do the same.

As many of you know, I'm involved in prison ministries, and the testimonies I hear so often have had the same theme of how people were away from God and then something terrible happened in their lives and they were brought to rock bottom and God saved them. God met them there.

I have a testimony, but it is totally different. It was difficult when this came, but there was no question in my mind, but that this was God's perfect will. I never asked why. When it was hard to take the next step I knew God would help me. He did. And when it came down to the day of the surgery itself, and I felt I couldn't take that next step, I just felt Christ pick me up and hold me.

A couple of hours before the surgery I was just weeping. The nurses probably thought I was a sissy, but I was just weeping for joy. For a couple of hours I was just thinking about God's blessing in my life and how He has blessed me.

A word of exhortation to you is: if there is any sin in your life, get rid of it; it's not worth it; it will interfere with your relationship with Jesus Christ. Just get rid of it.

Thank you.

****

I was a bit surprised by Dick's talk. He doesn't generally talk about himself like that, and I was expecting just the "thank you" part. The response to what he said was good, though, making me think that what he said was not just talking off the top of his head, but saying what God was leading him to say. I can only hope that Jeremy was listening to his father. Probably listening to his father's life story and hearing how Dick made decisions will be more helpful to Jeremy in choosing a college than any list of pros and cons that I can give him.

****

March 25, 1998

We met Dr. Busse, the radiologist, today. Dr. Bleday had told us that having a good radiologist is really important, because "if you shoot those rays in the wrong place, you can really get hurt!" We were somewhat surprised to find that Dr. Busse won't actually be shooting the x-rays, except for the first day, but he will be tattooing Dick so the x-ray technician will know where to "shoot" him.

We also had an appointment today with Dick's new primary physician – Dr. Michelle Coviello. It turns out that Dick has to switch his "point of service" in order to gain access to the group of physicians he wants to see in Boston. His former internist was only able to refer him to the oncologist, Dr. Huberman, as a one time second opinion visit. After meeting Dr. Huberman, we were definitely convinced that he is the physician we want to coordinate Dick's chemotherapy. He made me think of Einstein – with long white hair and great intelligence. He was also quite pleasant and <u>very</u> good about explaining things. He was very familiar with the protocols that the first oncologist had seen, but not used. So, there have been an awful lot of doctors' visits, but we feel quite confident that Dick will be getting the best possible care.

****

March 29, 1998

I've been having some sort of weird flashback-type experiences from some recent unsettling dreams. It happened a couple of times today. I can't really remember what the dreams were about, but I know that there have been several, and I think they have something to do with the cancer experience. I don't think the dreams were anything horrible, and though I can't remember anything specific, it is just unsettling. Maybe if I try to write down the dreams as soon as I wake up, I'll be able to get rid of this uncomfortable feeling about them.

****

March 30, 1998

I awoke this morning ready to record my dreams, but I couldn't remember anything specific. Thankfully, I didn't have any more flashbacks today! I am grateful to not be distracted by that because there are other things to think about.

Jeremy went to UVA for two nights last week and then went for a one night revisit to Webb. He loved the University of Virginia. He really likes the people at Webb, but says there is so much more to do at UVA. Also, he got a slightly different impression of the workload at Webb than he had the first time he visited. At that time, the students had just returned from a two month work-study program. This time they were more solidly into studying. He didn't visit <u>any</u> classes. I am quite astounded that Dick and I have spent about $650 for Jeremy to make these three college visitations, and with the four days he missed from school, he managed to visit only one junior level lab at Webb and walk through one studio class at UVA. He can't understand why I would want him to visit <u>classes</u> at college. "I know what classes are like. I go to school every day!" So much for really informed decision-making. Then there is Jeremy's most notable observation of UVA: "There are more beautiful women in one place than I have ever seen before in my life!"

The thought has occurred to me that if he goes to UVA, he might meet some beautiful southern belle, marry her, and then live down south closer to her family rather than coming back north near our home. I'd really miss him if he moved far away permanently, but I guess these thoughts are a bit premature! I should stick to living in the present - one day at a time.

Chapter 4

April 1, 1998

Dick's first two days back at work since the surgery went remarkably well, (though he said he spent a lot of time in the bathroom), but today he is exhausted.

****

April 2,1998

Dick woke up feeling as though he had been run over by a Mack truck. I figured something must be going on, so I checked his temperature: 100.4 degrees 45 min after Percocet and Tylenol, both of which should have brought his fever <u>down</u>. I paged Dr. Bleday, who wants Dick to come in. The doctor took a stool culture, but Dick looked so wiped out, that instead of waiting for the results, he decided to prescribe Flagyl for him right away.

****

April 3, 1998

The culture was positive for Clostridium Difficile: "C-diff". I don't know anything about this particular "bug", but the positive culture confirms that Flagyl is the correct medicine for Dick to be taking.

****

April 8, 1998

I returned home after being out for the evening to find Dick in great pain. He has been using the toilet a <u>lot</u> and now his backside feels raw. This pain is greater than I've seen him have. Dick says if he doesn't feel better by the beginning of next week so that he has a whole week of feeling good, he's not going to Cancun on April 20.

****

April 9, 1998

I woke up this morning feeling resentful. I know God will help me deal with it if we can't go to Cancun, but I don't understand it. The thought of maybe not going in addition to just the very idea of Dick's having cancer is more than I feel I should have to accept. Beside those big things, I have to deal with the reality of less important but irritating things like grubs. They destroyed our front lawn, eating away like cancer at the healthy roots of grass until the whole lawn, patch by patch, turned brown. Once again - for about the fourth time since we've lived here - we had to reseed the lawn. With all these issues, big and small, grabbing for my attention, my primary emotion this morning was resentment.

Now I knew I couldn't resent Dick, because he didn't cause any of these problems, and I couldn't resent God, because He has clearly been with us throughout this ordeal, so I ended up just feeling sad this morning. I was running around before work, trying to clean up the house, feeling sadder and sadder. I didn't want to burden Dick with my tears, so I went upstairs into the bedroom closet and looked out the window. I watched the crows and robins eating the new grass seed, and the tears came; no big sobs, just sad, resentful tears. However, I knew that as cleansing as tears are, I needed to do more than "let it out"; I needed to reach up. So I prayed. God knew I didn't have a lot of time to spare this morning, so He listened patiently and gave me a generous dose of PEACE.

****

April 14, 1998

I don't know if the C-diff is still there, even though the medicine to treat it is gone; I don't know if there is some new problem; and I don't know if Dick just hasn't healed from the surgery yet, but he's not feeling well at all, and the possibility of our going to Cancun seems to be decreasing. Today we tried all day to contact Dr. Huberman instead of Dr. Bleday, thinking that Dick's problem is medical, not surgical, but when Dr. Huberman finally called at 5:45, he said we should contact Dr. Bleday! We felt that the whole day was wasted.

At the supper table, I asked the boys which they thought was more important: going to Mexico, or being together as a family (a friend had offered to help care for Dick if we decided to go to Cancun without him.) I wasn't looking for a quick response, but Jeremy pretty easily replied that, "I think being together as a family is more important." Zach hesitated, but said that he agreed with Jeremy. What do I think? I don't know. I don't understand why God would bring us this far to let us down with regards to the trip, and I don't understand why He would have us just throw away $3500, but maybe that's something I need to learn: I don't need to <u>understand</u> God's ways; I just need to trust Him. I'm so tempted to try to figure out <u>how</u> God's ways could be better than the way I think things should be, but if I figure something out, that's probably not it either, because He is "able to do immeasurably more than all we ask or imagine." (Ephesians 3:20) So, I need to keep on with our "one day at a time" plan, nerve wracking as it is. A week from now, we'll either be in Cancun or we won't.

****

April 15, 1998
    With the ups and downs of reassurances and disappointments, life seems like a roller coaster ride. I hit another low point on the ride today. This morning I stood once again in the bedroom closet, looking out the little window, and cried. The closet is a good crying spot, since it is away from the active places in the house. I feel a little guilty that I'm trying to hide my tears from Dick, but I can't see how it will help him at all to have to deal with my frustrations and sadness as well as his own.
    He awoke with a fever of 100.0 and was unable to reach Dr. Bleday all morning. Dick went in to the doctor's office in the afternoon, but despite being started back on Flagyl for probable C-diff, his temperature went up to 102 degrees again this afternoon.
    The frustration that started for me this morning continued throughout the day at work and as I kept in touch with Dick by phone conversations. The aggravation peaked with a crying spell when my friend Jeanne stopped in to see me early in the afternoon. I was really grateful that it was she who was with me for the tears; I felt free to express my frustrations without fear that she would think that I was losing my faith. She knows that I really do believe that God is in control, but there's so much I just don't understand. I can't begin to imagine how the whole Cancun thing will turn out, and I don't even know how to plan. I truly want to do what God wants, but I just can't see how to figure it out. There are some verses in the Psalms: "Commit your way to the Lord" and "delight yourself in the Lord and He will give you the desires of your heart." I know that He can either give me the desires of my heart in the sense of granting my wishes, or He can create the right desires. It

doesn't matter to me which it is, but what do I do next? "Commit your way to the Lord." I think I'm doing that, but it is difficult to just quietly trust and not be anxious or angry.

Jeanne says it is okay to be angry with God. That's kind of a scary thought, but she says He's big enough; He can take it. I guess Job was angry, but he didn't curse God. That makes sense to me: that it is okay to be angry as long as one does not curse God.

I had a great revelation as I was driving home from work today: I've been trying to protect God! I've felt that I couldn't be angry with God, because He's done nothing wrong. I've also been careful in what I say to other people, lest they get a bad view of God. But God doesn't need my protection; He needs my adoration. He needs for me to delight myself in Him. I just wish I could figure out how to do that...

****

April 17, 1998

I put a call in to Dr. Bleday early this morning so he could call me when he was free. I made it a point to be near a phone all day - even taking the portable phone into the bathroom with me! By 7:00, I was pretty irritated with Dr. Bleday for not calling; with myself for thinking he would; with Zach for not eating his fruits and vegetables, and thus putting himself at greater risk for colon cancer; and with God, for not making His will about this trip clear. I had a few reasons for calling Dr. Bleday. I wanted to find out if the stool culture was positive to know if the medication that Dick is taking is the correct one. I also wanted to know if there is any reason why it would be unwise for us to take the trip to Cancun. Are there any other difficulties that might be expected related to the C-diff or Flagyl or surgery? Is there any preparation we could make for potential problems?

I might have maintained my irritation well into the evening, but it is amazing how quickly and easily anger can be diffused by just having something to take one's mind off the source of the anger. At 7:30 tonight, Sarah, Jeremy's girlfriend, came to visit me. Jeremy, who is working tonight, told her that she needed to stop by to check up on me to make sure that I was not annoying (!) Zachary and his new girlfriend, Olivia, who was planning to come here for the evening. Shortly after Sarah came, Olivia's mother Charlene drove Olivia here. I had never met Charlene before, but had spoken to her earlier in the day and

26

sensed that she was a bit anxious about this "date". "I'm a little nervous about Olivia liking a boy and having a boy like her," she told me.

As Charlene was backing out of the driveway in her white van, I heard a loud noise and realized that the van had hit the fire hydrant at the end of the driveway. This is a problem we have never had before, because we initially had a big bush by the hydrant, and for many years, after the bush was removed, the basketball hoop was parked next to it, so there was always something bigger than the hydrant that was visible when one backed out of the driveway. A few weeks earlier, we had moved the basketball hoop, so the hydrant stood alone, not high enough to be seen, but elevated enough to cause damage if hit.

Unfortunately, there was considerable damage to Charlene's car, though the hydrant remained unscathed. The fiberglass above the van wheel was cut and the tire was very flat. The scene became rather comical, with four women (Charlene, Olivia, Sarah and I) looking somewhat helpless. Dick was the man with the knowledge, and we soon enlisted Zach to be the one with the brawn. The tire finally got changed, despite Charlene's acute embarrassment, and along with the tire change, my mood managed to change as well.

****

April 18, 1998

We decided to proceed as though we are going on this trip to Cancun in 2 days, but we will be ready to abort plans right up to the last minute, if that seems necessary.

****

April 19,1998

We finally heard from Dr. Bleday! He said that the stool culture was negative for C-diff, but that false negatives are not uncommon. Since the Flagyl seems to be working, Dick should stay on it.

It seems that all we have been thinking about for the past few weeks is C-diff and Cancun, but the rest of life goes on as well. Jeremy has made his college decision: he decided to go to the University of Virginia (UVA). As a proud mother, I'm delighted to say that he also got into Yale, but he turned them down! (Too expensive.)

****

27

April 25, 1998

God is good. We went to Cancun, and it couldn't have been better. In all the confusion with Dick's health issues before we left, I couldn't understand what I was supposed to do or even what faith meant in this situation, but He worked it all out despite my uncertainties.

We stayed at a lovely resort with beautiful gardens, pleasant evening entertainment and plenty of good food.

The weather was <u>beautiful</u> and it was so very good to be together. The first day we rented speed boats to go snorkeling at a coral reef. The boating part was great for all the guys, but terrifying for me. On the way to the reefs, riding in a boat with Dick driving, I was sure I was going to pop out of the boat and die. I decided it might be safer for the return trip to ride with Zach instead of Dick, thinking he would be a slower driver, but those were groundless hopes. Do men have no fear? The snorkeling was <u>awesome</u>!

Another day, the boys and I took a one and a half hour bus ride to Tulum to see Mayan ruins, which were quite interesting, and we stopped to snorkel at a place called Xel Ha on the way back. Dick decided to just relax at the hotel instead of taking the long trip.

Each evening we were there, after the hotel entertainment, we enjoyed playing cards together. Dick was very careful about what he ate the whole time we were away, and he had no medical problems. That in itself was a huge blessing!

God's goodness was certainly evident throughout that wonderful trip, but after four days of fun in the sun, it's hard to be back to the rush, rush, of our normal routine: laundry, soccer games, meal preparation, etc.

Tonight I went to a youth worship gathering at church. It was a really good time of worship, but I spent most of the time at the back of the sanctuary (packed with hundreds of kids) crying - being reminded of God's holiness, grace and faithfulness – and realizing that not only is vacation over, but I am about to start on a totally new phase of life - full of unknowns. Thankfully, Carolyn was there to offer her support.

Hailstorm:

April 1998 - July 1998

Chapter 5

April 27, 1998 - In the oncology department
I took the day off to accompany Dick for what may be his first day of chemo. He needs blood work done and then to be "randomized" for the clinical trial (of chemo and radiation.) He may start chemo today.
We found Dr. Huberman's office without difficulty, but we have had a long wait, because they have just moved the whole office to a different location and Dick's medical information got lost in the computer shuffle. Nonetheless, he got his blood work done and was examined by Dr. Huberman, who is trying to gather the necessary reports to proceed with the randomization.
Sitting here in the waiting room again, while the doctor determines if the chemo will start today, I find myself not wanting to look around too much. This is a very busy place, and though everyone is very warm and friendly (they even have ex-cancer patient volunteers giving out juice and donuts), it's hard to not think about the reason we're here. There are a couple of wheelchairs, but most people get around on their own. One redhead across the way looks healthy, but her hair is obviously a wig. Several people wear scarves or baseball hats. Most are here with a friend or relative. How is Dick going to fare through all this? Will he be weak? Lose hair? Need someone with him each time he comes?
Today I had more of those uncomfortable dream flashback things. I don't like them!

****

May 3, 1998
The first week of chemo went fine – just a little nausea, controlled by Compazine – but here were are, Sunday am – back in the ER with what sure feels to Dick like C-diff again. Dick felt lousy yesterday, but no fever until this am - 100.6 - when he awoke. I called Dr. Koon - the fellow on call for Dr. Huberman. Since Dick just had the week of chemo, the doctor feels he needs to have blood work done - especially to check his white count.
I sure wish there was something that could be done about this C-diff. I don't know that C-diff is the cause of the fever and discomfort, but the symptoms are very similar to those he had before with that infection.

30

The whole cancer experience, with the surgery and treatment, is long and arduous enough without Dick's feeling so sick so often. This morning he said he'd like to "pull the plug." Sigh. I think one of the hardest parts of all this for me is when he feels not only sick, but depressed as well. Mostly he's been great; he sure has <u>reason</u> to be depressed, but I haven't seen much of it. Still, it's hard when his spark dies down.

In the midst of hard times, I appreciate the moments of normalcy in our lives: working, having Dick work, monitoring the boys' activities, meals together. I need to really live those moments fully because when I think how rapidly my life is changing, it's easy to become overwhelmed. I've often liked to look ahead and think of what <u>might</u> happen in a given situation to be prepared for it, but it's too hard to do that in my life now. I find I need to <u>assume</u>, for example, that the chemo/radiation will go according to schedule and that Dick will be feeling okay following a month of rest in August and be able to drive with me when we need to bring Jeremy to school in Virginia. If something changes, I'll deal with that at the time. One day at a time.

I can reason these things out logically, but I'm not doing very well right now with "delighting myself" in God. I <u>believe</u> in Him, I <u>appreciate</u> Him, I <u>love</u> Him, I <u>trust</u> Him, but I'm not <u>delighting</u> in Him. I am not sure exactly how to do that, other than spending time with Him, in His Word and in prayer, and I'm just not making that time now. I need to . . .

Dick's blood work came back normal, and the doctors are waiting for the results of a stool culture. They will meanwhile assume that the problem is C-diff again, and treat him accordingly – with Vancomycin this time. Turns out that this is a very pricey drug: it would cost us $452 for one course of treatment if it weren't covered by insurance!

Even though I'm not doing well with "delighting myself" in God, I'm grateful that the boys seem to be doing well dealing with Dick's illness. A few weeks ago, Zach gave the devotional (a little message that the students give) at a youth group meeting. I came late to the meeting that night, so I missed it, but apparently he got up and said that his dad had been sick, and when I came home from the hospital, he knew it was bad, because I was crying. He reportedly spoke of a real peace that he felt in God and read the passage in the Bible about God taking care of the lilies of the field, and how much more He cares for us. His sense of peace and his strong faith were a real encouragement to me at the time – and still are.

31

THROUGH THE BARREN TREES

****

May 4, 1998

Detached, tired, numb, defeated, accepting, helpless – all words which could describe my emotions by the end of today. I'm a little puzzled that I wasn't more upset by the events of the day, but detachment was more practical, I guess.

Our friend Rick drove Dick in for his CT scan and appointment with Dr. Huberman today. I probably would have been better off taking the day off. Instead, I got to deal with one of the ultimate joys of elementary school nursing: finding three girls with head lice!

At the end of school, I made what was supposed to be a quick trip to the travel agency to straighten out a mistake with Jeremy's airline ticket (for coming home from college at Thanksgiving.) It ended up getting further confused and ultimately costing 50% more than the original ticket.

I returned to school for a staff meeting, arriving after the meeting had started. There was a guest speaker talking about (of all things) stress management. She had some good ideas, but I felt that the potential effectiveness of her suggestions would be limited, since she proposed that we look <u>within</u> rather than <u>up.</u>

I couldn't reach Dick when I tried to call him from school before I left, but I decided to stop at the supermarket for a few things ($146 worth). When I finally got home about 6:00, Zach greeted me with the news that Dick had a problem. He'd had a difficult time with the CT scan, and had been vomiting and having diarrhea and gas pains since he got home. Since he couldn't reach me, he had called Rick to come back to take him to the hospital to be admitted. Dr. Bleday is away, but Dr. Stone, who is covering for him, says there might be a leak in the anastamosis (where they sewed the colon to the rectum after removing the cancer.)

Since I got home before Rick arrived, I drove Dick in – tough long ride, but Dick was kind enough to comment that it was a "smooth ride." He was admitted to the hospital and started on IV antibiotics. He will be given no food by mouth for a few days and be kept under observation to see if the "pockets" (abscesses?) near the surgery site heal. If not, the more aggressive treatment is surgery: either inserting a needle through the buttocks to drain the abscess, or else a temporary ileostomy to allow the rectum to heal completely. Neither of these options sounds great, but I'm feeling rather detached about the whole thing - or maybe I've just resigned myself to being powerless.

32

By the time I left the hospital tonight, Dick was feeling a little better, despite having been poked and prodded by a number of people. Since Beth Israel Deaconess is a teaching hospital, there are often medical students and interns and residents as well as primary physicians who do examinations.

****

May 7, 1998

I'm sick of all this: pain, running, rain, fatigue, uncertainty. I want it to be over now! But it <u>always</u> happens – even with the Great Flood: after the rain comes the SUN. Sometimes it takes awhile, but it <u>will</u> come out again - in the sky and in my life. Meanwhile, all this rain is really good for the grass, which is finally growing. It's quite patchy in spots, but patchy is workable; it looks pretty good from across the street.

I guess my life feels "patchy" too; some areas are certainly "green" but there are barren spots where the germinating grass is not yet visible. Friends are so kind, but even phone calls are beginning to feel burdensome. I come home after visiting Dick in the hospital and invariably there are several phone messages from people calling to see how we are doing. I don't usually have the energy after a long day to call back, and if I do, then I get to bed too late to get a really good sleep.

We talked with Dr. Bleday today. He explained more about Clostridium Difficile (C-diff). It is apparently found normally in about 2% of the general population, and 30% of the health care population, or people like Dick who are in the hospital so much. It doesn't normally cause any symptoms, but when someone has antibiotics for abdominal surgery to prevent infection, the antibiotics kill off the <u>good</u> bugs that usually keep the <u>bad</u> bugs like C-diff in check. C-diff needs more powerful antibiotics to kill it.

****

May 8, 1998

Tonight is Jeremy's high school prom, and he has been very busy with preparations. I have felt that it is really important to him, so I wanted to be home to share his excitement and help if needed, but when I asked him a question, he interpreted it as my still thinking of him "as a 5 year old." My fragile psyche crumbled under his rejection of my well-meant overtures, and I dissolved in tears - not exactly the kind of support I had

33

wanted to offer. Jeremy was very supportive and apologetic, and after I cried for a while and he offered to vacuum, our conversation became a bit more productive about his post prom plans.

I had another couple of crying spells after my discussion with Jeremy; I just want Dick to be home and not sick! After taking pictures of Sarah and Jeremy, Zach and I went in to the hospital. The news was pretty promising: one of the doctors reported that the two tests that Dick had today looked good. The inflammation around the incision site has decreased, and the pocket has apparently shrunk and is not connected to the anastamosis. Therefore, he thinks Dick can eat solid food for breakfast and then go home on oral (pills) antibiotics.

****

May 9, 1998

Dick was discharged today. He got lots of rest, but we also went to see Jeremy's art work display at the town library, and then we bought a grill, which Zach assembled. It is <u>very</u> good to have Dick home!

****

May 10, 1998 – Mothers' Day

Although I haven't felt I've been a great mom lately, and thought I deserved <u>nothing</u> for Mothers' Day, all my men got up to make me a wonderful breakfast and shower me with gifts. It was the things that came from the heart that were so special: Zach's pressed flower wall hanging (with flowers from Dick's hospital bouquets) and Jeremy's card: "Happy Mothers' Day Mom. If anyone deserves the best, it's you. *Inside:* That's why you have <u>me</u>!" He wrote a note, too: "I know I treasure the relationship we have and I wouldn't trade it for anything. You're not only my mom; you're one of my best friends, too."

****

May 12, 1998

"I feel great!" Those words were music to my ears! Dick reported - before I was even out of bed - that he was down to 150 pounds (he had been holding at 155-160), but he felt great, so was going off to breakfast and then early to work - maybe to come home early to nap before supper and the National Honor Society induction.

34

****

May 14, 1998
I'm sure grateful for some "ups" between the "downs". The honor society induction was an up. Mother's Day was an up. Tonight is a down. Dick's temperature is UP again (101). That is a down. How could it be up when he is on "enough antibiotics to bankrupt a third world country" as Dr. Huberman said? At least Dr. Bleday returned Dick's call tonight (up) and said we should just "watch" (down). Sigh.

Kim - the teacher from school who also has colorectal cancer - came in to work today to see her students. It was one of her "good days", but I saw her at the end of the visit and she was clearly tired - very thin, poor color, and wearing a continuous morphine drip pump for pain control. No one said it, but it is obvious that she is dying, and when I think that she has the same disease as Dick... It's hard.

****

May 19, 1998
I went to an oncology nurses' seminar on colorectal cancer last night. It was encouraging to hear that Dick's treatment plan is really the best of what is being done today.

Part of my life change right now is that I can no longer focus on plans and dreams. I've always enjoyed that, but things are much less sure than I used to think they were. I don't know how Dick will respond to treatments, so any plans that are made may need to be broken or changed. That's a bit hard for me, because one thing that is important to me is being with friends, and sometimes Dick is just too tired for that.

Then there is Jeremy's anticipated leaving. Yesterday morning Dick said he'd had a nice breakfast with Jeremy on Saturday - "just the two of us. I had a chance to say good-bye. I wanted to do it not at the last minute with all his friends around. I told him that all his life so far we'd been building towards this point and that we are very proud of the way he's turning out."

GOOD-BYE?!?!? Just the word brought me to tears. It sounds so permanent. I know he's leaving soon for camp for the summer and then college, but the thought of actually saying good-bye is just too painful.

****

May 30, 1998

Despite continuing to have a fever (never greater than 101 degrees) for the past two weeks, Dick has been working - full time except for chemotherapy or doctor's appointment days. He tires easily, but we've still had some good family times, such as suppers together at home and Sunday lunches out at restaurants.

Last weekend was Memorial Day weekend, and the boys (initially at my suggestion) decided to do something together with their girlfriends. Their plan, initiated by Jeremy, was guaranteed, he said, to earn them "major points" with the girls. (It did.)

Jeremy and Zach started their preparations in the morning - making chicken cordon bleu and rolls from scratch. The first batch of rolls could have doubled as hockey pucks, but the second attempt came out great. The girls, Sarah and Olivia, arrived, dressed up, at 6:30 as instructed, and were greeted by Jeremy and Zach, respectively, decked out in jackets and ties and each bearing a single peach colored rose. Jeremy had typed the dinner menu, and the table was set - complete with lace tablecloth and candles - on the porch. They had sparkling cider and grape juice and non-alcoholic sangria and the girls were served their custom made salads first and then the rest of the meal by their handsome waiters. Dick and I, of course, were not allowed to be part of all this (though I must say that my supervision for the preparations was invaluable!) We barbecued on the deck, but did each manage to take a stroll around the yard and peek casually into the festivities on the porch.

It was a successful evening.

Kim died on Monday. It was really sad at school. She was such a bright light and such a fighter. I went to the wake on Wednesday after school. I think half of the town knows her family. People have been very solicitous of me - knowing that I will be thinking about Dick since Kim's diagnosis was the same - yet not quite. Both were apparently Stage III cancer, but Kim's cancer was visible outside the colon during surgery, and Dick's was not. I have not wanted to make comparisons to Kim all along, but I have sort of had to: had to be glad that Dick's cancer isn't so bad.

Dick started his second round of chemo on Tuesday (May 26), but Wednesday when he had to cross the street to bring a stool specimen to Dr. Bleday's lab, he ended up arriving for the chemo a little short of breath. His temperature was 101 degrees (again) and the medical people finally decided to take notice. (It seems they had to actually see this fever - which has been off and on now for two weeks - to believe it.)

Anyway, they took blood cultures and checked his blood oxygen level and decided he should have another CAT scan. They did that Thursday, and it showed a whole mass of infection - like a sponge - around his coccyx (tailbone), which has been hurting for over a week. Dick was exhausted by the time he got home Thursday night, but he went to work for the morning on Friday anyway, knowing by this time that he was going to have to go back in for surgery on Monday to clean out the infection. Jeremy took him in for the chemo yesterday, and I made arrangements to take off Monday. Today went we went in for the chemo (on a Saturday because of the holiday last Monday.) It went well, but Dick was just feeling so rotten - not really wanting to eat much, and wanting to drink even less - that the nurse and I decided to call Dr. Bleday, who wanted him to be admitted today instead of waiting until Monday.

I came home for a while and then the boys and I went in to visit Dick. We played Pitch, a card game that Dick had taught us, and he won both games. He looked perkier than he did earlier in the day. I'm glad he is there.

Our twenty second anniversary yesterday was uneventful.

****

June 1, 1998

I arrived at Dick's room today just as they were preparing to take him down for surgery - a couple of hours earlier than originally planned - so it's a good thing he was already there! They let me go with him to the prep room, but kicked me out after a few minutes. I got home about fifteen minutes before Dr. Bleday called to say that the surgery went well. They flushed out the infection with antibiotics and he has a drainage tube in, which, if all goes well, should come out Friday (four days from now.)

Tonight Dick is feeling great - "the best I've felt in a long time" - thanks to his "happy button" (my affectionate name for the button he has to self-administer his morphine when he needs it.) I told him I'm glad he didn't use drugs when he was younger or he'd probably still be getting high since he enjoys feeling good so much! He was so cute today - repeatedly telling me that he loves me.

****

June 5, 1998

What a joy to have Dick back again - not only home, but back to his "old self." They discharged him at 9:00 PM Wednesday night (June 3), but he still has the drain in and a "mid-line" for intravenous medications. A visiting nurse came last night to do the first IV med and show us how to do it. It's a once a day medication to go through next Monday, June 8. Things are so different since I worked for a Visiting Nurse Association; we didn't do IV meds at home. Anyway, I just did it tonight, and it really wasn't a problem.

Dick looks and feels so much better than at any time previous to this since the surgery. I guess that infection was really keeping him down.

****

June 7, 1998

Jeremy's graduation this morning was <u>great</u>. Grandparents from both sides of the family had come for his party yesterday, along with other relatives and friends, and we continued the celebration with a very pleasant family brunch on the deck this morning before leaving for the ceremony.

We arrived for the outside graduation - at the high school football field - in plenty of time to get good seats. It sprinkled just before graduation and again when it ended, but we stayed dry for the one and a quarter hours of the ceremony. We couldn't have been more proud of Jeremy as he gave his salutatorian address. He spoke about the future and how success must not be measured by material things but by contentment in being true to who you are. He ended with a quote (which my friend Jeanne had given to me and I had passed on to him): "If we do not have within us that which is above us, we shall soon yield to that which is around us."

38

Chapter 6

June 8, 1998

Today felt rather anticlimactic after all the excitement of the weekend. I felt <u>really</u> sleepy all day, and Dick felt lousy. He saw Dr. Bleday, who took the drain out (even though he had said he would not take it out until it was producing less than an ounce a day, and it was still draining more than that.)

Dick's arm was quite sore from a phlebitis (inflammation) at the IV site. Although Dr. Bleday had said earlier that I should give Dick one more dose of the IV antibiotic and then take out the line, he instead called the visiting nurse to come and take out that line and start another line just for the last dose of medication.

All of this medical stuff happened early enough in the day that we were able to go the Underclassmen's Award Ceremony at the high school for Zach. That turned out to be a <u>huge</u> pick-me-up, as Zach walked away with <u>four</u> gold medals (given for the student with the highest grade point average in each subject for the year) and he also received the Outstanding Freshman Award! He is such an individual: when he got the first medal, he was quite surprised, having only anticipated one or two silver medals, and he sat down wearing the medal. Most students remove the medals when they sit down, but he chose to keep it on. When he went up for the second medal, the two medals clanged together a bit, eliciting some little snickers from the audience.

At this point I said, "Most people take the medals off when they go up again."   "Well, I'm not," he replied.

So, there was more clanging and laughter when he went up for number three. After that, he apparently decided that there had been enough clanging, and he went up for the fourth medal with only his tie around his neck.

Men. They can be wonderful and they can be such heartless creatures. This morning I was praying and feeling sad as I thought about Jeremy leaving tomorrow for camp for the summer. Dick came down to fix his breakfast as I began to cry, so I figured I could get a bit of comfort from him in the form of a good hug. I went up to him as he was pouring his milk on his cereal, and he put his arm lightly on my shoulder. I figured his arm was hurting from the phlebitis, and after he finished pouring the milk, he would give me a big hug. Wrong. When he finished pouring, he started eating! I left him, muttering a few choice words under my breath, and went off to have a good (short) cry by myself, before realizing the humor of the situation and returning to call him a heartless soul. In all fairness, he was as sweet as could be later in the day, saying he hadn't realized the gravity of the situation.

****

June 9, 1998

Today Dick had his appointment to be marked for the radiation treatment. I didn't go with him, but his description of the experience made me unhappy (and since Jeremy left for camp today, I was already feeling a little "down"). Dick's appointment was a bit disappointing for several reasons. In the first place, he didn't see Dr. Busse at all, and my understanding was that this was the one time he would see Dr. Busse, whose expertise was reportedly needed to assure that Dick was "marked" correctly. Besides that, Dick said that the technicians were not particularly gentle or empathetic. One of the most disheartening occurrences, though, was a comment he had from the doctor that he saw today. The doctor pointed out that while "you're doing the right thing" (having the radiation treatment), the radiation can, in fact, cause cancer in 10-20 years. We had gotten the impression earlier that the future looked pretty good if Dick could make it for five years cancer free.

Another big discouragement today is that Dick's tail bone is starting to hurt again and he feels generally lousy. Could the infection still be there?

****

June 10, 1998

It was clear that we had to call Dr. Bleday again this morning. Dick has that old wiped-out feeling again. He got up for his shower, then lay down again; up for breakfast, then down again. Dr. Bleday's response, when Dick filled him in on his current status, was that he was looking for an antibiotic that would specifically treat the "bugs" that Dick has, and he feels that Dick should have another CAT scan. He also said "it might be time to involve the infectious disease people." Sure sounds like a good idea to me!

After waiting all afternoon for Dr. Bleday to call in an antibiotic to the pharmacy, we finally reached him by paging him. He identified the "bugs" as Klebsiella (which responds well to many oral meds) and Proteus (which does not.) When I asked if it might be time to insert a central line (a longer lasting sort of IV line which goes into a vein deep in the neck), he agreed. He had already talked with the infectious disease people, and it really seems that using IV meds is the only way to go. Dr. Bleday will insert the central line for Dick tomorrow.

****

June 11, 1998

Sometimes getting appointments arranged can be reasonably straightforward, and sometimes it can become an exercise in communication skills and patience. Such was the case as I tried to find out the time for Dick's central line insertion today. We knew that we were supposed to report to the Day Care Unit on the eighth floor of the Farr Building at the Deaconess Hospital, but we didn't know what time, so I decided to call them directly.

Call #1 - To Deaconess Hospital main number

Nancy: Could you please connect me to the Day Care Unit?

Operator: No, you have to dial that number directly. The number is 617 . . .

Nancy: Thank you.

Call #2 - to the above number

Person who answered: Child Care

Nancy: I'm trying to reach the Day Care Unit

Person: This is Child Care. I can't help you.

Call #3 - To Deaconess Hospital

Nancy: Could I please have the Day Care Unit - not Child Care, but like Day Surgery

Operator: Certainly

Transfer made to Call #4

Person who answered: Same Day

Nancy: I'm Nancy Kline and my husband Richard is supposed to meet Dr. Bleday there today for a central line insertion and I was wondering what time it's scheduled for.

Person: I wouldn't know anything about that. This is Same Day Surgery. You'll have to contact the Day Care Unit.

Nancy: Yes. Could you please connect me to them?

Person: One moment.

Transfer made to Call #5

Person: Day Care Unit
Nancy: Hi. I'm Nancy Kline... (as above)
Person: Oh, I wouldn't know anything about that, but you could talk with the nurses.
Nancy: Yes, please.
Person: Hold on. I'll transfer you back there.
Transfer to Call #6
Person: Nurses' Station.
Nancy: I'm Nancy Kline... (etc)
Person: Well, I haven't heard anything about that, but you could talk to Cindy. She's in charge.
Nancy: Thank you.
Transfer to Call #7
Person: Hello, can I help you?
Nancy: Is this Cindy?
Person: No, Cindy's not in.
Nancy: Well, I'm Nancy Kline...
Person: I really don't know anything about that. You'll have to call the doctor's office.
Call #8 - To Dr. Bleday's office
Nancy: Hi. I'm Nancy Kline, and...
Person: Actually it's Cindy who arranges all that. I'll call over to her and have her call you.
Nancy: Thank you.
Waited 15 minutes. No call from Cindy.
Call #9 - To Day Care Unit.
Person: Day Care
Nancy: Could I speak to Cindy please?
Person: No one named Cindy works here.
Call #10 was to Dr. Bleday's office
Call #11 was a call back from him to finally get it set up.
I am glad that I am able to see the humor in exchanges like the one I just recorded. It would be rough if I only saw the aggravation and not the humor! My emotions have been fairly stable lately - though honestly much more up than down. Having the surgery seemed like a real solution to the infection problem, so that was an "up"; and Dick was discharged sooner than expected, so that was another "up". Then he seemed so good for a few days: it was like we had the old Dick back. Graduation (and the party) and Awards Night were major "ups". I was acutely aware that just as we don't "deserve" the hardships of Dick

42

having cancer and difficult infections, so we don't "deserve" to have two extremely bright, nice, handsome boys. Nonetheless, this very resistant infection is quite discouraging. I am sure that God can use all this to teach me something(s). I hope I'm listening enough. What I have heard so far is:

 1 - Delight in the Lord - first - above all else. (I'm still working on this.)

 2 - Take one day at a time.

 3 - Make plans, but don't count on your dreams or plans.

 4 - Appreciate the little things. (That's not a new lesson for me.)

 5 - Make the most of each moment (easier at some times than at others.)

 6 - Worrying is pointless and wastes lots of time and energy.

 7 - There are lots of people in my life who really care!

 8 - What some might consider "little" expressions of caring (cards, flowers, help with activities, a caring comment) really have a big impact. (I'd like to practice this more towards others.)

 9 - God's timing is amazing - incredibly good. For example: giving us "ups" when they are most needed.

****

June 13, 1998

 Dick's mother also is apparently experiencing God's grace in a significant way. This is part of a letter we just received from her, dated June 10.

 I phoned Dick and told him of the very special "experience" I had when I finally realized that no amount of my worrying was going to help him, that it was in God's hands, and I felt this great weight and ache lifted from my heart and mind. It was such a wonderful feeling of peace. I am still maintaining that feeling of peace and I am sure that, together with the new medication my doctor has given me, I will not be having any more severe angina attacks. I fully realize that the best thing I can do for those who love me is to stay as well as possible - which I intend to do.

 So much for the good news. Despite being on the IV antibiotics for two days, Dick still wasn't feeling much better, so I kept a close eye on his temperature, which spiked again to 102 degrees at 11:00 last night. I prayed a lot last night that the fever would go down, and the infections would clear, but especially that God's will would be done and I would have the grace to accept it. Part of the grace came in the form of my good friend Bobbie Converse's offer to drive us in to the hospital tonight. Dick's temperature had gone down a bit this morning, so he went out to breakfast with the boys, but he was tired and in pain when he arrived home. He slept most of the day, but when the fever continued despite another dose of antibiotic, we called the doctor who was covering for Dr. Bleday this weekend. Once again, it was decided that he needed yet another CAT scan, but the torrential rains today made me really hesitant about driving into Boston again. Bobbie's offer was a real godsend, because the roads were flooded in some places. Dick was admitted to the hospital again, so I was glad to not have to drive home alone.

****

June 15, 1998
Email from me to several friends
Subject: Dick's health

Hello from the Klines! Many thanks for all your prayers. We certainly feel the love of many friends and God's sustaining grace at this time. We've had some great times in the midst of Dick's ups and downs - the trip to Cancun and Jeremy's graduation weekend (as salutatorian!) as well as many other fine, though less dramatic family times.

Jeremy left last Tuesday for a summer job as a lifeguard at Camp Berea in New Hampshire, but came home again Friday night to take his life guarding test on Saturday. Thankfully, he passed. He'll probably visit home occasionally during the summer on his days off, making the separation a little more gradual than it will be when he leaves for the University of Virginia at the end of August.

So much for the good news. Dick is still in need of much prayer and encouragement. He is in the hospital again (for the third time since his original surgery.) This is all because of a persistent infection, which apparently has been present since the surgery, but which is getting more difficult to fight because of his depressed immune system due to the chemotherapy. He had surgery to clean out the infection on June 1, but it came back immediately after his IV antibiotic was stopped. Currently he is having high fevers, and his white blood cell count is quite low, so he expects to be in the hospital until the fever goes down and the white cells go up. We'd like to think that this will happen soon.

Meanwhile, he's a bit discouraged about not being able to work. He had thought that this period of time (between the surgery and the radiation) would be the time when things would be nearly normal, but that he might be tired during the latter part of the radiation. Though he's had some (quite a few, really) good days of work, it hasn't been nearly as consistent as he would have liked.

On the plus side again, he is feeling a bit better today than yesterday, and the white count seems to be slowly climbing. School will be out for me in a week, so I'll be more available. At least all this is happening in the good weather, and not in the dead of winter.

So, that's the update. Sorry it is not more personal to each of you. We do appreciate you!

Love,
Nancy

****

June 18, 1998

It is now day six of this current hospitalization. Dick has been on "neutropenic precautions" because his white blood count dropped quite low (1.8, when it should be 4-10) and his neutrophils went down to 400 (they should be at least 1000). The precautions mean that he is in a private room, and people have to wash their hands before going in and take other precautions so that Dick is protected from other people's germs, since he doesn't have an intact immune system to fight infections. At the beginning of the week, his temperature spiked twice to higher than 103 degrees, but it has been staying reasonably low for the past few days. When he was first admitted, the doctors felt that they had to check every possible source of infection, though it was generally accepted that the infection was in the same place as it originally had been: near the tailbone.

Blood counts have been improving; last I heard, the white count was 4.1 and the neutrophils were up to 800, but meanwhile there seems to be a cold war going on between the doctors, and I think Dick is getting caught in the crossfire! The ID (infectious disease) guys are now involved, though apparently a bit "put out" that they were not called in sooner. Dr. Bleday and the surgical guys, on the other hand, seem less than enthusiastic about the input of the ID guys. Meanwhile, there is really no one coordinating Dick's care, since his primary care physician is out on maternity leave, and he only met her once in her office anyway. I feel as though I'd like to have a tea party and invite all these doctors to come and talk together about the best plan for Dick. He seems content to follow Dr. Bleday's recommendations, but it is frustrating when those recommendations at times seem directly opposite to those of the ID guys!

Today Dick had surgery again because - at his own suggestion - the doctors took another look at the surgery site to make sure there was no leak. Lo and behold - there <u>was</u> a leak! Last night a surgical resident had explained the anticipated procedure to Dick, but the explanation he got from Dr. Bleday this morning sounded quite different to him. Dick had been extremely hopeful last night in anticipation of this "fix it" surgery, but he sounded confused and much less optimistic this morning. I suggested that he might want to have a better understanding of the surgery before signing the consent forms, but he responded that "they're the experts" and wouldn't hear of further discussion. I felt so helpless - not comfortable with going ahead with the surgery without better understanding it, but having no recourse <u>to</u> better understand it. All I could do was call Dick's nurse and ask that she talk to him - but without saying that I had called her, since he hates it when he feels I am too pushy. It is very difficult to be an advocate / helper but at the same time to be limited by Dick's opinion of <u>how</u> I should advocate.

Sometimes, he does find my presence helpful when talking to doctors. One time an infectious disease doctor asked Dick if he had been out of the country recently and he said "no", so I reminded him of the Cancun trip.

The same doctor, who had a heavy Greek accent, also asked, " Do you have any pets?" Dick stated that we have a dog, and the doctor asked, "Does your dog 'leek'?" "No," Dick replied, "he's well trained; he goes outside." It occurred to me that maybe the doctor was not asking if the dog had a problem holding his urine. When I asked the doctor for clarification, it turned out he was saying, "Does your dog <u>lick</u>?" !

When Dr. Bleday called me after the surgery today, I was dismayed to hear that there was still major disagreement between the ID and surgical doctors. One ID guy felt that the infection had gone into the tailbone, and that therefore Dick should be on IV antibiotics for 5-6 weeks. This fellow "saw" the infection on the x-ray, but none of the other doctors did. Dr. Bleday felt that a tailbone infection was very unlikely, and that therefore the long term antibiotics were not indicated. I, on the other hand, felt that if the infection <u>might</u> be there, why not treat Dick as if it is, and keep the antibiotics going? Dr. Bleday later came in while I was visiting Dick and said that the ID guys are "dragging their feet" about deciding what antibiotics to continue for Dick. They, on the other hand, were expecting a culture from this procedure today, but Dr.

Bleday said a culture would have been useless because it would have had stool in it. Boys, boys, boys!! Let's just all work together, shall we?! Dr. Bleday described the procedure he did today to allow the infection to drain so the rectal area will heal over the next few weeks. Right now, after this last conversation with Dr. Bleday, I am finally feeling less angry. It was easy to be angry when I did not understand things.

I have not reserved my anger just for humans; I have also been angry with God - maybe not angry so much as disgusted - but then, I quickly reject that word. I'm certainly not disgusted with God, but I just feel disgusted, helpless, angry: Job-like. I wonder if perhaps Satan is wandering now (like he did in Job's day) looking for some righteous people to afflict. I don't feel all that righteous, so I don't know why he would choose me, but things seem to go from bad to worse with this infection that has afflicted my dear husband. Even the good little things that have always given me a boost seem to be overshadowed by irritations. The rain is one such irritation; it has a way of falling - hard - at the most inopportune times. It rained for the last five minutes of my ride in to the hospital yesterday and for my walk from the parking garage; and today it rained just for my walk from the parking garage. There are irritations at work as well. This morning it took me at least six tries to get into my computer program at work, and kids kept coming in to my office with issues that really did not require the assistance of a nurse. I do seem to have difficulty focusing on the good things of life lately; I am actually having some difficulty finding them so that I can focus on them.

I have also been thinking about the issue of prayer and how it relates to my faith. My faith in God is quite intact. In thinking about Dick's infection, I reasoned that if all these very educated, highly experienced doctors could not all together figure out one part of one human's body, how could people possibly think that the human body just happened - that there is not an infinite Creator God? The body surely points to intelligent design. Anyone would say it is ludicrous to imagine that a few wires and some metal and plastic got together and formed a computer, yet people consider the complexity of the human body and still say there is no God. To me, this is illogical, and I am more convinced than ever that God exists.

So my faith in God is intact, but my understanding of and belief in the importance of specific prayers has surely altered. We have prayed repeatedly for Dick for healing from this infection. I've prayed for good weather for traveling. I've prayed that I would be able to care for Dick while continuing to work, without feeling overly stressed. God has said, "no, no, and no." I know that God, for our own good, sometimes answers, "no", but I'm at a place where I often do not see the point in praying specific prayers, because obviously I'm praying against God's will, and that's certainly pointless. I should be able to see and remember that sometimes the specific prayers are answered with a "yes" (like Jeremy passing both his life guarding and his water safety instructor courses) but when I'm in the middle of "no's", my field of vision becomes rather narrow, and I forget the "yes's" that are not right in front of me.

****

June 22, 1998
Changes happen very rapidly for Dick these days. Saturday, two days ago, he could hardly get out of bed. Yesterday he was discharged, and today he went back to work! He is on IV antibiotics again - three times a day. His temperature stayed below 99 degrees all day!

****

June 24, 1998
Dick received this Father's Day Card from Jeremy. Father's Day was this past Sunday.
Sorry this is a little late - there's not a lot of places to buy decent Father's Day cards up here. I had to wait until I had a half a day off to go to Concord. Anyway, enough said about that. I just wanted to take this opportunity to write some things that have been on my heart lately. I know that I have never been able to express myself as clearly to you as I can to Mom - maybe it's my male pride needing to keep a tough exterior in front of my father. Anyway, I know I can write what I need to say. First, I need you to know the admiration and respect I hold for you. The older I get, the more I see the realities of the world and realize what a special man you are: God shines through you in everything you do and interact with: work, family, and even leisure time. You have done a magnificent job with our family, giving us a sense of security which I am just now learning not to take for granted. As I grow, I can only strive to pattern myself after you and everything you stand for. As I compare the man you are and the man I am becoming, my short comings become that much more evident. Even though I have never been able to express it as much as I feel, I need you to know that I love you more than I can describe. You are the ultimate role model for a young man to aspire to.

48

Finally, I need to express the guilt I feel at not being there for the family this summer. I feel that in this present case of your temporary sickness, I need to be the man of the house, yet I cannot be there for the family. I know this is where God wants me, but it is still hard. I pray for your healing every day, because I still need you, as do many. Thank you for being such an awesome Dad.

Hopefully I'll see you soon. I love you!

Love,

Jeremy

Dick commented that "this is the card that every father hopes to get someday from his son, but he doesn't really expect it until maybe his son is 35 or 40 years old and has his own children and begins to realize how much he appreciates his own Dad." He felt very privileged to get this from his eighteen year old son.

Chapter 7

July 1, 1998

This time Dick was home for almost a week and a half before he went back for his fifth hospitalization and fourth surgery in just under four months. Last week started out quite well. Dick worked shortened days; he went in a little late and was home by three or four o'clock each day for his medication. By Wednesday night, however, after having diarrhea all week, he started to feel ill again: tail bone pain and very slight fever. He lost some of his appetite and was not inclined to drink much, so by Friday morning, when he stood, he felt lightheaded. I checked his blood pressure, which stayed rather low until Saturday, when the doctor on call for Dr. Bleday ordered increased IV fluids for the next several days. The fluids helped the blood pressure, but the tail bone pain worsened.

Meanwhile, Zach left last Saturday for New England Frontier Camp in Maine. We had intended to drive him, but decided it would be wiser to have him drive up with Bobbie, who was going up to work as camp nurse. We made plans to visit Zach next weekend.

When we finally spoke to Dr. Bleday on Monday about all Dick's problems - diarrhea, fever, and especially the pain - it didn't take him long to suggest that we proceed with what had been a possibility in the first place, but hadn't really seemed necessary at the time of the original surgery: a temporary ileostomy. This should allow the rectal area to heal and the infection to clear completely. Dr. Bleday also suggested that the ileostomy not be closed until at least a month after completion of the chemotherapy and radiation, since both the chemo and radiation could hinder healing.

At 10:00 this morning, Dick had an appointment with Paula, the stoma nurse, for some teaching prior to the surgery. She was very clear and helpful in explaining things, and although she welcomed my participation in the discussion, she made it clear that I will not be the one doing the ostomy care; that will be Dick's job. Of course that made sense; I've never helped him with going to the bathroom before, and ostomy care will be what he does instead of going using the toilet in the typical way. Nonetheless, I was just a little surprised that she was so adamant about Dick doing the ostomy care alone, because I have gotten so used to the role of caregiver while taking care of his intravenous line and medications.

50

We met with the anesthesiologist today shortly before the surgery. I was glad to have that meeting because Dick has had so much trouble in the past with intubations. This anesthesiologist was able to speak with the one who had done his last two surgeries and learn from her experience. When I spoke with Dr. Bleday after the surgery, he said that the anesthesia went very well, as did the surgery itself. Another positive report he gave was that although Dick "is presenting as a chronically ill person", there was no sign of cancer in the abdominal cavity. He feels that he needs to be built up nutritionally due to his weight loss and his low hematocrit and hemoglobin. He suggested that Dick take chewable children's vitamins - like "Flintstones" - since they will be absorbed better than some of the adult vitamins.

****

July 2, 1998

Dick never did come up to the room when I was waiting last night. Jeremy came to the hospital about 7:00 PM, and at around 7:15, he asked if he could go to the recovery room to see his dad, since he had to leave soon for New Hampshire (to get back to camp). We were given the "okay", and found that the reason he had been in the PACU (Post Anesthesia Care Unit) so long was that he was having trouble with pain, so he was using a lot of morphine, which was depressing his respirations. When we saw him, he was quite perky and reported to us that he was having trouble remembering to breathe, so he was on a respiratory monitor. He described the problem to us in great detail: "I forget to breathe and the beeper goes off and it goes BEEEP BEEEP BEEEP, but my mind doesn't connect that that means I'm supposed to breathe, so the nurses call, 'Breathe, Richard, breathe!' and I breathe." By the time we saw him, the pain was better, but he still needed a lot of reminders to breathe. He was really glad to see us. He took Jeremy's floppy hat and put it on his own head and looked quite comical with the funny hat and tubes attached all over him. Dick told Jeremy that he was very proud of him and loved him. I'm glad Jeremy got to see his dad before going back to camp.

Later in the evening, Dick was transferred from the PACU to a Step Down Unit, where there was the possibility to keep him on a monitor and there was also a better nurse: patient ratio than he would have had on a regular floor. He stayed there until this afternoon, when he was transferred again to a nice private room.

****

July 3, 1998

I called Dick's mother last night. She said she had been really "down" - apparently thinking about him and feeling sad that "such a good man" had to go through all this.

Today the reality of the ileostomy seems to be hitting Dick. He is most distressed by the sound it makes - much louder than he had thought it would be and quite unpredictable. He's concerned about how he will be able to be in public with it. I suggested that Dick might want to talk with someone who has an ileostomy (the stoma nurse had suggested this) but he is reluctant to do so. It's not his style to talk with people he doesn't know, and he figures that the person he would meet might have a personality that is different from his. Therefore, he feels that the other person's suggestions in dealing with ostomy problems would not be helpful. Dick figures that another person couldn't <u>eliminate</u> the problems such as noise, so there would be no point in talking with him. Sigh. I wish he would at least be open to looking at how to <u>deal</u> with problems that may not be able to be eliminated!

I felt lonely tonight. Both boys are away, and our good friends are out of town for this holiday weekend. I talked to Dick about my wanting to go to the Night Before the Fourth fireworks display, and he suggested I call Barbara, the mother of one of Jeremy's friends. I did, and she invited me to a cookout with some neighbors and friends of hers. She said she had been thinking of calling me, so that made me feel less like a party crasher. After we ate, we went to a place where we had a great view of the fireworks. I'm glad I took Dick's suggestion. It was a good reminder that people are kind and caring.

Another example of the kindness of people was a couple of weeks ago when Jeremy and Zachary's eighth grade science teacher called. He said he had just heard about Dick's illness and wanted to offer what help he could. He paints houses in the summer, so he has tall ladders, and he offered to come to our house sometime in the fall to clean our gutters of leaves. What a thoughtful, concrete offer!

****

July 4, 1998

Yet another drive into the hospital today - so many traffic lights! I counted them once - 28 each way. At least this time I got to bring Dick home. I'm afraid I wasn't great company for the ride since I was in a rather bad mood from some confusion about medications at the time of discharge, and Dick felt nauseous just before he left. Sometimes I wish he would be kept in the hospital longer to make sure that everything is okay before he leaves. Also, it is tough discharging him on a holiday weekend when homecare is involved. At least today Dr. Bleday was on call, so I paged him when we got home and he was able to answer quite a few questions for me.

When I get in a bad mood or frustrated, like today, sometimes I think: What's the point of life? I don't feel at all suicidal, but life seems so meaningless sometimes. You do the same things over and over - and for what? Just to do them again. Take cooking and eating and cleaning up for example. You do those things, and then you have to do them all again - over and over. It's the same thing with cleaning the house, or going to work - or anything! What makes up a life? You are born, then you grow up, go to school, get a job, get married, have kids, have good times and bad times and then you die and your kids grow up and go to school and get a job and get married and have kids and have good times and bad times and then they die, too. I know I'm going to Heaven, so sometimes I think it would be nice to just skip the earth part. I shared my thoughts with Dick, and he reminded me that it is not God's plan to "skip the earth part." I pondered what I know of God, and concluded that He made us for a purpose, and as far as I can understand, that purpose is to worship Him and to bring others to Him.

So since that is the plan and that is my job, I guess I had best accept it and do it. I must not think of my life as pointless, because that is sort of like a slap in the face to my Creator. Bad analogy, but if I were to spend a lot of time and effort making a beautiful gourmet chocolate cake, and the cake decided to explode itself because it didn't want to exist because it thought, "What's the point? I'm going to get eaten later anyway," I'd probably, as its creator, be rather unhappy. That cake, in its short existence, could really perk someone up, and that would make me happy. In the same way, I must remember that my Creator did make me for a purpose, and it is not helpful to bridle against that purpose.

Even as I am beginning to work through the issue of my existence and purpose, the reality of life at present is that Dick's treatment is going to be a really long haul. We originally thought that the six months of chemotherapy and radiation would be long, but workable. The delays from the infection stretched out the treatment and recovery time, but now, with at least six months for the ileostomy, the picture has really

53

changed. I've tried to tell myself that the ileostomy is no big deal, but in fact it is. There are dietary modifications that need to be made, and many more fluids that need to be ingested (and this is not easy for a man who does not like to drink.) There is the issue of the noise from the ileostomy, the fear of dehydration, the threat of blockage if he eats the wrong foods, and in the background, the concern about whether the infection and the leak in the anastamosis are going to actually heal. I was feeling really grateful today that it is summer and therefore so much easier to make the trip into Boston, but it looks like this all may drag on well into the fall and even winter.

Okay. So that's all out. Facts are facts. It is my choice how to respond to them. I need to take my own advice. It is a lot more pleasant to be around me and I feel a lot better if I choose to view my glass as half full rather than half empty (even if sometimes it seems it is only a quarter full!)

****

July 5, 1998

Okay. I think maybe I am starting to understand. It seems that this summer could be kind of a drag: no vacations to plan and look forward to; the boys will hardly be here at all; waking up at 6:00 - 7:00 each morning after less than 8 hours of sleep to give IV meds and knowing that this could go on for a long time if there is a bone infection; many, many more trips into Boston; watching my husband be in pain, both physical and emotional; etc., etc.

So how do I turn that around so it doesn't look so negative? Well, I could remember that some people have it a lot worse - like Christopher Reeve (the actor who became a quadriplegic when he was thrown from his horse) and his wife; or that everybody has his or her problems; or I could go back to remembering that there is a purpose to my existence rather than just to exist. The Bible commands me to "love the Lord your God with all your heart" (Deuteronomy 6:5) and "love your neighbor as yourself" (Leviticus 19:18) and exhorts Christians to "present your bodies as living sacrifices, holy and pleasing to God - which is your spiritual worship." (Romans 12:1)

So the purpose of my being here is to worship with my life - the things that my body does each day - and those should be acts of love. Therefore, each time I get a drink for Dick, or wake up to give him his medicine, or drive that long road into Boston for an appointment or to see him, that is not only an act of love for him, but an act of worship, which is why I am. There may be fun times along the way - times to laugh or things to look forward to - but I need to start viewing each positive act I do - cleaning up the house or whatever - as an act of worship. That must be the essence of me. Of course, it is only by His grace and with His help that I can do this, but if it is truth, it's possible!

****

July 11, 1998

Dick came home one week ago today. There has been a lot of progress in a week that did not start out well. Monday he had another CAT scan; that was a bad day. He could take nothing by mouth after midnight Sunday night, and when he felt nauseous upon rising on Monday morning, there wasn't much he could do about it. By the time we walked from the garage to the hospital, he was ready to vomit - mostly dry heaves - but after drinking the contrast solution, he really had something to vomit, and he did. Poor guy.

We saw the ostomy nurse, Paula, after the CAT scan, and she made a good attempt at being encouraging. Monday afternoon was a little better, and each day Dick has improved a bit - though slowly. He's really making an effort to drink more. Lemon-lime Gatorade and vanilla Ensure Plus seem to go down the best. He continues to be tired, but unfortunately has been unable to fall asleep for the past two or three nights.

Thursday Dr. Bleday removed Dick's central IV line. We decided to postpone the radiation and resumption of chemotherapy for one more week to allow Dick time to get his body built back up and to feel better.

Toward the latter end, we are taking a little break today. We are at Cape Cod, staying at a cottage belonging to my generous friend (the head school nurse) Cathy. The cottage is a lovely, little, very newly renovated four room place called "Honah Lee", located just 7 houses from the beach. What a gift to be able to stay here!

Meanwhile, Jeremy stopped by home this morning on his way to Connecticut for Sarah's cousin's wedding. The stopping had two purposes: 1 - to see Dad, and 2 - to leave off his laundry. Just before he arrived, I decided to check some things he had received from UVA to see if there was anything that needed to be addressed soon. Sure enough, there was something from the School of Architecture which had to be returned no later than June 26! He must have opened it just after graduation and then ignored it. He did complete it and Dick mailed it, but I'm sure that there is more that needs to be done in preparation for college. I sometimes worry about his priorities; is he really ready to be off on his own?

While I am a little concerned about Jeremy, we got a really nice phone call from Dick's mother. She was excited because she realized that Dick is in <u>God's</u> hands and not hers. She got this insight after reading about Shadrach, Meshach and Abednego in the book of Daniel - how they were thrown into the furnace but were not burned. I guess a lot of us are learning things through this illness.

****

July 18, 1998

We just ended a <u>wonderful</u> week. Dick worked full days every day this week and the fever and pain did not return! Ray and Elizabeth arrived Thursday from Africa to begin a three week trip of visiting colleges and friends. Today we also picked up Zach at camp. He has had a great three weeks. It sounds as though he has had some really solid discipleship training and very good, creative learning experiences. When I asked if he had had any "a-HA!" learning experiences about his faith, he cited the importance of <u>love</u> in all his actions. Great lesson!

I had a very encouraging conversation today with Becky, the cook at New England Frontier Camp, where Zach has been. I was reminded of God's supernatural provision for us. Becky and I had enjoyed talking with each other on several occasions in the past two summers when I spent a week at camp as camp nurse. We did not keep in touch with each other, but about two months ago, for some reason she started to think about me quite frequently. Shortly after that, she heard from our mutual friend Bobbie that Dick had cancer, but she knew no details about his complications. At that point, about five or six weeks ago, she started to have very strong urges to pray for me; she would actually see my face, and my name would flash before her mind. As I look back, that would have been just about the time that Dick was at a very low point physically - hospitalized for the infection and low blood counts. Hearing of her prayer for us makes me think that this illness has been more than just a battle against cancer or infection. We believe that it is a spiritual battle, and the forces that God has amassed in His army are quite remarkable!

56

****

July 21, 1998

Four days ago I got my ear pierced - again. This makes hole #3 for the right ear. I got the first holes when I was 40 years old and the second set when I was 45. It hasn't been 5 years yet, so why did I do it now? I think Jeremy is probably right; he said it was a "wild and crazy" thing to do. I expect that I've just had too much time of being responsible lately, and I needed to do something a bit zany.

Dick started radiation today and resumed the chemo. He has continued to feel well and have no fever. The IV pole and supplies have been removed from our home, and we have had several basically "normal" days, including having lots of people around. After the first radiation treatment and a chemo treatment, we went to dinner at the Addis Red Sea Ethiopian restaurant in Boston with Jeremy, Zach, both their girlfriends, Jeremy's friend Pete, Ray and Liz. It is always an interesting experience eating there. The first time we ate at an Ethiopian restaurant was in Nairobi, Kenya. The boys like Ethiopian food so much that we found this restaurant a bit closer to home. The restaurant patrons sit on low chairs around small round tables. Food is ordered for the whole party, rather than for individuals, and is served in piles on a stretchy bread called enjira. Using extra pieces of enjira as well as what is under the various dishes (lamb, chicken, beef, vegetarian - flavored hot or mild), one rips off a piece of the bread and scoops up some of the other food. It is a much more community style of eating than that to which we are accustomed. We had a most enjoyable time.

Ray was quite impressed that Dick would be willing to be included in the above adventure, having just had his treatments. Ray says repeatedly that he is amazed at Dick's and my response to this whole illness experience. His feeling is that because of what we have learned in the past in our faith walk, we were prepared for this occurrence and have appeared to take it in stride. I have assured him that we have had our share of tears and frustrations, but he seems to think that there is strength in our overall attitude and outlook.

I agree with the idea of "preparation" for this time in our lives. Some of that preparation for me began a year or two ago on a Sunday. The fellow who was leading the singing in church said, "Do you ever wonder what God's will for your life is?" That caught my attention, because it seems to be a constant question for me. He then gave the answer from the Bible in 1 Thessalonians 5:16-18: "Be joyful always; pray continually;

give thanks in all circumstances, for this is God's will for you." It surprised me that it was stated so clearly and concretely. It struck me that this was something that I could actually practice: being joyful, prayerful and thankful. I typed up these verses and put them on the refrigerator and my bedroom mirror and in the bathroom and on my bulletin board at work, and I have been making a concerted effort to heed them.

In the recent months of upheaval in our lives, I am very grateful for "breaks" such as this past week has been. God has provided several "breaks" since Dick first became ill: Cancun, graduation weekend, and now this past week of time with family and of Dick feeling quite well. Although Dick and I hope for a least a few good weeks during radiation, we recognize that there will most likely be struggles, but at least we are able to start with his feeling healthy.

****

July 29, 1998

Dick continues to do well; he has now completed seven of twenty-eight treatments - one quarter done! He has had occasional slight nausea; Oreo cookies seem to help eliminate the nausea. That's not what I would have expected, but whatever works is great! I went in with him for his treatment today for a change of pace, but he has been going in on his own every day since that first day last week. He has no chemo this week or for the next two, so he is able to get to work and work about two-thirds of each day.

We are back to a quiet house again. Last Wednesday, Ray and Elizabeth left to look at colleges, and Pete and Jeremy went back to camp to continue their work as lifeguards. On Sunday Dick and I drove Zach to New Hampshire for soccer camp at Keene State College.

I had some trouble again a few days ago with those flashback things (I don't know what else to call them). It happened while I was preparing breakfast Sunday and I actually felt light-headed and sweaty. I had the same physical response once again when I was consciously trying to think of the dreams to identify and deal with them. As far as I can recall, the dreams are not bad or frightening in any way - just uncomfortable. I talked to Dick about them and he thought that it could be a psychological thing and that it might be good to visit a Christian psychologist; maybe it is not an uncommon phenomenon for someone dealing with stress. His second thought was that it could be spiritual - an evil or demonic sort of attack. He described an experience that he had had with this many years ago. I decided that the most prudent (and cost effective!) course of action would be to start with the assumption that the problem was the latter of his two suggestions, so Monday morning I prayed in the name of Jesus that if this was a demon, it would be gone. I have had no more trouble, but I am also aware that I need to make a conscious effort to keep my mind occupied with "whatever is true, noble, right, pure, lovely, excellent, admirable or praiseworthy", as it says in Philippians, rather than thinking about those dreams to try to figure them out. I am very certain that this is not some past trauma coming back to haunt me (since I have had no past traumas!) so it is basically an annoyance. Certainly as Dick is doing well and I am truly excited about God's provision, Satan would love to find some way to knock me down a few pegs. Nice try, but the Bible says that "greater is He who is in you than he who is in the world." Very reassuring!

Partly Sunny:

August 1998 - December 1998

Chapter 8

August 5, 1998

It was such an encouragement Saturday to be at both New England Frontier Camp (dropping Zach off again) and at Berea (visiting Jeremy) to hear very good reports about both boys: to have people say how well they are doing. We stayed at Berea Saturday night after taking Jeremy out to supper and then went to the worship service at camp on Sunday. It was quite moving for me, having the camp director share that people at camp had been praying for Dick since the beginning of the summer and were very glad see him there, looking well.

It is interesting to look back now - from a good place in terms of Dick's health - back to when he just wasn't getting better because of the infection, and we really wondered why our prayers weren't being answered or what the point of specific prayers was. Now I see it as the "Footprints in the Sand" story describes it. The story talks about a man walking along the beach with God, leaving two sets of footprints. However, in looking back over his life later, the man notes that during the most difficult times of his life, there is only one set of footprints, and he questions why God would abandon him at those critical times. God responds lovingly that during those difficult times, He did not abandon the man, but instead He carried him. We are well aware that during our most difficult times, God was definitely there for us.

Jeremy asked last weekend if he could spend his whole paycheck for one week instead of saving half of it as we had agreed at the beginning of the summer. Apparently he had found a great study Bible that he really wanted to buy, and he wanted the leather version, because he figured he would have it for the rest of his life. He also wanted to buy a pocket version of the Bible so that he could carry it around with him. Permission to spend the entire paycheck was granted!

It has been four weeks since Dick's last surgery, and he has had no signs of infection. He continues to work two-thirds of each day, and radiation is going well, with no significant side effects. Since things are going so well for him, and so well with the boys, it is almost hard to believe how much we were "in the pits" just a little over a month ago.

****

61

August 12, 1998

Ray and Elizabeth have come and gone again - this time back to Africa. Between all our visiting with people and watching many videos with Dick, I have been reading When Bad Things Happen to Good People, by Rabbi Harold Kushner. The book was given to me by someone who had read it and found it encouraging - as have many other people - but I am finding it to be disturbing and sad. Reading it at this time, having just struggled with the very issue it addresses, I find myself coming to some very different conclusions from those of the author. While we share concern over the obvious "unfairness" of some of life's occurrences, and we share a belief in the existence and inherent goodness of God, my sadness comes because it seems to me that the author has a small view of God. His god is not all powerful, did not create the world out of nothing, and does not have ultimate control in the world. Someone once presented the idea that life is like a tapestry of which we humans only see the mass of apparently meaningless threads on the underside, but of which God sees the beautiful picture from the top. Kushner rejects this idea. He also, I think rightly, rejects the notion that pain and evil are caused by an individual's sin, but from what I have read in the first half of the book, he apparently gives no thought to the notion of original sin, the fall of man, and the entrance of evil into the world.

He acknowledges God's availability and willingness to help the sufferer, but he appears to equate justice and fairness. To my understanding, these last two words are not equivalent. God is just, meaning that He does what is right or righteous, but He is decidedly not fair. If He were fair, then I would be punished for my sins and He would not have sent a Redeemer for me. If He were fair, I would not have all the blessings I have in my life: wonderful, bright, handsome, God-fearing boys and a faithful, gentle, bright, understanding husband who loves me. No, God is not fair, and it is a good thing for me that He is not!

In an effort to explain the difficult things in life, the author concedes that sometimes there is no reason for bad things happening, but he chalks that up to chaos in the universe that is left because God did not quite finish creation, which, in his interpretation, was fashioning order out of chaos. Either that, or there is "residual chaos" over which God has no control.

I, on the other hand, do not feel it is necessary to try to explain those things that are difficult to understand. I am sometimes saddened, and sometimes angered, and sometimes confused, but I am left with a picture of a God who is not less powerful than the world's chaos, but so much bigger than my finite human mind can comprehend, that I, having experienced His unfair love, can accept His omnipotence and wisdom. I can accept that He is way beyond my comprehension, and that is all right with me!

****

August 15, 1998

I am continuing to enjoy reading When Bad Things Happen to Good People, finding that it is sharpening my thinking and clarifying my beliefs. I still agree with some of the author's notions, but find some others sad, lacking a true appreciation of the fullness of God. In his chapter entitled "God leaves us room to be human," he conjectures that when God said, "Let us make man in our image," the "our" referred back to previous verses and meant the image of animals and God. I'm not sure if he is saying that animals participated in creation (let us make...) or just that he believes in evolution. He points out that the difference between us (humans) and animals is our freedom to choose.

Later on in that chapter, he talks about the Holocaust, wondering why God did not intervene - striking Hitler dead or demolishing the gas chamber by an earthquake. He says he has to believe that God

"was with the victims, and not with the murderers, but that He does not control man's choosing between good and evil. I have to believe that the tears and prayers of the victims aroused God's compassion, but having given Man freedom to choose, including the freedom to choose to hurt his neighbor, there was nothing God could do to prevent it."
(Kushner, When Bad Things Happen to Good People)

Is this last phrase what he means when he says that God is not all powerful? If it is, I still reject that notion, because it is God who gave us free will, and therefore has the power to remove it, should He so choose.

Interestingly, I very much agree with the quote with which Kushner chooses to end this chapter, and with which he apparently agrees. It is a fair summary of my own conclusions, but was written by a Holocaust survivor.

"It never occurred to me to question God's doings or lack of doings while I was an inmate of Auschwitz, although of course I understand others did. . . I was no less or no more religious because of what the Nazis did to us; and I believe my faith in God was not undermined in the least. It never occurred to me to associate the calamity we were experiencing with God, to blame Him, or to believe in Him less or cease believing in Him at all because He didn't come to our aid. God doesn't owe us that, or anything. We owe our lives to Him. If someone believes God is responsible for the death of six million because He didn't somehow do something to save them, he's got his thinking reversed. We owe God our lives for the few or many years we live, and we have the duty to worship Him and do as He commands us. That's what we're here on earth for, to be in God's service, to do God's bidding."

(Brenner, The Faith and Doubt of Holocaust Survivors, as quoted by Kushner in When Bad Things Happen to Good People)

****

August 29, 1998

Change HURINS! We just left Jeremy off at UVA. Intellectually, I know this is a good thing; we've raised him to be independent and to someday go off on his own, but why today? Why now? Why not in another five years? When I think of his chomping at the bit and chafing under our control, and when I think how well he did this summer at Berea, I know it's the right time and even the right place, but gosh I miss him! I'll even miss sharing the hotel room with him tonight.

My friend Arlene said it was horrible leaving her daughter Hayley at college, but she refused to talk about it. I understand now. I didn't want to cry when we said good-bye to Jeremy at the car. I was so hot and sweaty that I thought there were no tears in me, but I couldn't help letting a few fall. I was glad for my dark glasses and I put on a real forced smile; I'm sure it didn't fool Jeremy. After we hugged, he accepted a ride to the next street corner (UVA is a huge place, and we had already done a lot of walking.) I was okay when he got out, but not for long.

I figured I would come back here to the hotel and have a good cry in the shower, but I have never been one who could turn the tears on and off. They most often come quite unbidden, as they have since I got out of the shower. Dick is trying to find a place to eat. I am not very hungry. What I really want to do is leave right now and go home as fast as we can to be with Zach again. I don't even want to go back down the main street towards UVA to find a restaurant; irrational, I know.

Everything leading up to the final moment of separation actually went quite well. Jeremy came home from camp for a few days before we headed down here to Virginia. He had some good visits with his friends, but I wanted a little family time before he left. When his friends kept dropping in all day his last day home, I informed them that visiting hours

64

in the packing zone were limited - sort of like in an intensive care unit - and they all took it pretty well when I kicked them out. We did manage to have a very nice brief family prayer circle on the deck. (I kept my emotions in check then.) Jeremy did all the driving after we left Thursday afternoon, including driving through New York City. Dick was clearly exhausted by the time we stopped for the night at about 1:00 am. (Jeremy and I knew he must be really tired, since he was willing to pay $110 for the night at a Holiday Inn). He admitted today that he had felt really lousy yesterday, but felt greatly improved today. I am really glad Dick came. Today was hot and busy, unloading Jeremy and getting him settled and attending introductory meetings at the School of Architecture.

Jeremy seems ready for this phase of his life. He seems to have a reasonable amount of trepidation about college (minor), but not the stress we saw when he entered middle school or high school. Also, Berea was a good stepping stone for college. It was a time for really strengthening his faith and convictions. Nonetheless, leaving him was so difficult for me that it makes me conclude that the pain of childbirth is just a preparation for the pain of separation when a child goes to college!

****

September 13, 1998
Email from Dick to several friends
Greetings to Charles, et. al.

First an explanation concerning the above salutation. Charlie left a voice mail on our answering machine indicating that he tried to contact us and was wondering how we were doing and asked that I update him via email. This is the update Charlie requested, but it occurred to me that there have been many people praying for us, and it is difficult to remember who we have talked to and / or emailed when and who knows what. Therefore, I thought that I would write a general update letter and send it to all. For some of you this information may be redundant due to previous recent communications, but hopefully you won't mind.

Let me start out by saying the past two months have been good (praise God) and that at present I am feeling good (mostly). As most of you know, the months of April, May, and June (thereabouts) were difficult months, mostly due to a recurring infection. I was not feeling well much of the time during those months, returning to the hospital multiple times (5 hospitalizations and four surgeries), being treated for the cancer the first time, and for the recurring infections on subsequent hospitalizations,

65

returning home for a week or two, and then returning to the hospital again.

During this time we were very cognizant of the many prayers that were being offered up on our behalf, but for a long time it seemed like God wasn't listening. I can remember feeling almost apologetic to people that they were praying so faithfully for us, but I wasn't getting better; indeed, it seemed like I kept getting worse instead of better. It was very difficult during this period to keep telling people that I wasn't getting better.

I was originally supposed to start the radiation therapy in mid June, but the radiation was postponed because of the infections until mid July. The last surgery turned out to solve the problems with the recurring infections. The last surgery was an ileostomy, which if required at the beginning of all this would have probably devastated me, but at that point, I was willing to try anything that would help make me better. The ileostomy was successful in that my temperature returned to normal and the infections did not return.

By mid July I was feeling much stronger and was ready to resume the chemotherapy (which had stopped for a month) and also start the radiation treatments. This was the six week period that "they" had verbally prepared me for at the beginning of all this to expect to feel sick, especially by the end of the radiation period. However, I tolerated the radiation quite well. In fact, I gained 18 pounds during the time of radiation (most people lose significant weight during this period), gaining back the weight I had lost during the infections. I had some external radiation burns and some internal pain and cramping near the very end, but nothing severe. I finished the radiation treatments about two weeks ago, and the side effects have mostly subsided by now. I'm feeling stronger every day, pretty much back to feeling my normal self.

I have two more rounds (months) of chemo and will then be done with my treatments. After that I will need one or two more operations to basically undo the ileostomy, and possibly to redo the resection of my large intestine.

I'm feeling great and looking forward to the day when this will be behind us. However, we continue to feel truly blessed by God and continue to feel overwhelmed with His faithfulness. Much of that comes from realizing the number of people who are praying for us faithfully. We have also seen that God is in control of our calendar. Throughout this summer there were several special events that we really wanted to attend, which included a family trip to Cancun, Jeremy's graduation from

high school, attending Katie Ludwig's wedding, and the car trip to Virginia to deliver Jeremy to the University of Virginia where he is a first year student. God was faithful in that we didn't miss a single event. I was up on my feet and truly feeling good enough to enjoy each one. Thank you all for you prayers, love, and concern.
Dick

Chapter 9

September 19, 1998

   I have largely recovered from the separation trauma of leaving Jeremy at college. Clearly the trauma was mine and not Jeremy's. Despite a bad throat infection (some weird bacteria that was treated with penicillin) he told us on the phone that "if I'm having this much fun and I feel this bad, then college is going to be great!" His computer also died just after he got it back from having his Ethernet card (for email) installed, but he seemed to take all these problems in his stride. We've been appreciating the ease of email communication; in some ways it is superior to phone conversation, because each party writes only when he or she feels like communicating. Sometimes Jeremy is not available when we call, or he may not feel like talking, but when he emails us, he offers some news. It sounds like he is starting off with a good balance of fun ("Virginia League" soccer, watching football games), friends and studying.

   For my part, I am getting used to being a family of three. The "just three" now feels different from how it did when Jeremy lived at home and went out with his friends, leaving three of us for supper or the evening. It actually is easier now to deal with his absence than it was before he went to college, because before if one person was missing, I really wanted that person with the rest of us, but now three is okay because Jeremy's supposed to be away at school. One good side effect of Jeremy's being away is that Zach and I are having more fun together. Zach has been in Jeremy's shadow for a long time, but it has been fun in Jeremy's absence to spend more time with Zach and communicate a little better and just fool around together.

   Dick continues to feel well. He is so back to normal that we even got a bit irritated with each other a few night ago! He starts chemo again next week for the first of his last two months. We don't know yet when he will have his CAT scan to determine if his anastamosis leak has healed. Once that is determined, he will have more surgery. For now, he feels well and life is good.

****

Dick and I asked if we could each speak for a few minutes at our church on Sunday, September 20, 1998 (his forty-eighth birthday). After thanking people for their prayers and filling them in on his medical status, this is what he said:

But through it all, one thing I want to say is: we are really convinced that we are in a spiritual battle. During one of my five hospitalizations, I read through the book of Job, and I just saw the cosmic battle that was going on with Job: what was going on in heaven.

I was humbled, because I said, "Who am I? I'm just an ordinary man; I'm not a biblical personality such as Job," and yet we were convinced that the battle was going on in the heavens. One of the reasons was because we were so amazed at the reports that continued to pour in about people praying for us - not just locally from the church here. From Amherst Massachusetts we heard how my testimony affected people out there. In New Hampshire and Maine, many people were praying for us. In several different churches in Connecticut, Tennessee, Virginia, South Dakota - even as far away as Romania and Kenya - people were praying for us.

We just became convinced that something very special was happening. We were also amazed by the number of people who said to us, "We are praying for you every day." There are even two women from another state who are praying and fasting one day a week for me during my entire time of treatments.

During the three months that the infections were there, it was a rather humbling experience because so many people were praying for us, and yet for so long I wasn't getting better, but worse. At those times I almost felt guilty because I wanted to be able tell people that their prayers were being answered, but it just didn't seem like they were at the time, even though they have been now.

During this difficult time I was working with the young adults here at church. We were studying Daniel and one of the things that really struck me was when we read Daniel chapter 10 which is in the prophecies of Daniel. Daniel was a righteous man. He was probably in his 70's at this point and he had been reading in the book of Jeremiah and realized that the end of the captivity was coming.

He really wanted to know what was going to come after that, so he prayed and fasted and yet no answer came right away. That was difficult for him. Finally an angel came to him and brought the answer after a considerable period of time:

"Then behold, a hand touched me and set me trembling. Then the angel said to me, 'O Daniel, you are highly esteemed, understand the words that I am about to tell you and stand upright, for I have now been sent to you ... Do not be afraid, Daniel, for from the first day that you set your heart on understanding this and on humbling yourself before your God, your words were heard, and I have come in response to your words. But the prince of the kingdom of Persia was withstanding me for twenty-one days; then behold, Michael, one of the chief princes, came to help me, for I had been left there with the kings of Persia. Now I have come to give you an understanding of what will happen to your people in the latter days.'" (Daniel 10: 10-14)

So his answer came, but I was surprised to read that God heard right away and sent a messenger right away, but it took a period of time for Daniel to get his answer because there was a great battle going on.

I don't really understand prayer. I know God has the power to heal me instantly at anytime, but I also know that God has a better plan. I don't always understand it. He allows evil to battle against goodness in this world. He allows evil to battle against goodness in the heavenly realms.

I think the important thought that I would like to leave with you is just to say how important it is to know God: to know His love, to know His goodness, to know His compassion, to know His very character. If you know Him, you can make it through almost anything.

I spoke after Dick, also thanking people for their prayers and concern and for being available for us, and then I shared some of the lessons that I had learned and recorded in my journal. I was very prepared for my talk - I had typed notes and had gone over them - but when I listened to the tape of the service later I was quite disappointed. I've always thought that my voice sounds terrible on tape (not at all as it sounds to me!), but I was also surprised to hear how fast I was speaking. I've had some hidden aspirations to be a humorous motivational speaker some day, but that tape effectively squelched those dreams! Nonetheless, several people said they appreciated that we had spoken.

****

November 9, 1998
Email from Dick to friends

Dick here! I'm feeling good. I finished the radiation treatments around the end of August and I finished the last of the chemo injections two weeks ago, although this is considered a chemo month in that the effects of each chemo treatment peak about two weeks after the treatment (i.e., about now). Blood counts drop which results in some weariness, but I'm doing fine.

I've been fighting an ear infection the past week (maybe the result of low white blood cell count?) making me feel like a two year old, but it seems like that too is going away during the past 24 hours.

Still facing one or two more operations to perform some reconstruction. Not sure yet how many or when; should be having some tests soon and meeting with the surgeon to discuss. My best guess is mid-December?

Jeremy loves UVA. The three of us went down to Virginia to visit Jeremy on Columbus day weekend. Although he had only been there a little over one month, he said that it felt like home to him. That was met with mixed emotions by us, especially Nancy.

Even though we have had some difficult times, we continue to be amazed at God's blessings. For me personally, I have really become aware of just how precious each day is. Although, now that I am truly getting better, I find that the every day "rat race" is creeping back into my life. But I'm trying not to forget just how precious each day is.

Love to you all,
Dick

****

November 29, 1998
Email from me to Ray and Jan

It's been very good to have Jeremy home for Thanksgiving break. The house has been a much busier place for the last couple of days - lots of his friends coming and going - including Pete - his friend from Berea that you met - who came Friday night and left this afternoon.

God has a way of giving just what we can handle - in the big things and the little things. Here's a little things example: I purchased Jeremy's plane tickets for Thanksgiving last MAY- in order to get a good price and to get him on the plane with the guy who was going to drive him from UVA to Dulles Airport in DC. There was a little snafu with the travel agent booking him on the wrong flight, and when she corrected it she charged me a SECOND $10 fee, but I forgave that at the time. I've just taken the forgiveness back, however, because they apparently CANCELLED Jeremy's reservations for both ways, despite the fact that

71

we PAID for the tickets and HAVE the tickets (except for the time when they were lost in the mail for about 2 weeks that we DIDN"T have the tickets, one of which was sent by certified mail, but for which I LOST the certified mail receipt, but only for a time, and then after he GOT the ticket, I FOUND the receipt.) Okay, so about the CANCELLATION. He had his ticket in hand to come home, but when he got to the airport they said that his reservation had been cancelled, but they got him on the flight. So, today I figured before he left for the airport, that I'd better confirm his flight, but it COULDN'T be confirmed because the airlines said the travel agency had CANCELLED the reservation on NOVEMBER 4. What's more, the airlines wasn't about to reinstate the reservation, because they had no PROOF that he had come home on the flight on which he came home. The agent CHASTISED me because he didn't save his BOARDING PASS from that flight (!!!) Well anyway, "long story short" as they say, I became irate, irrational, irritated (3 good ir words) and told the agent that I was DUMBFOUNDED (dumb word, but that's what I said) and gave the phone to Jeremy. Somehow, she finally accepted that he was on that flight and gave him a seat assignment. So he's gone - not on the plane yet, but hopefully will be.

So anyway, that whole little snafu was a little easier to handle because I'm not particularly stressed at the moment (at least I <u>wasn't</u> stressed.)

Academically, Jeremy seems to be doing well - working hard and really loving architecture. He LOVES UVA.

Zach also is working harder than he would like to be working now. Regarding a current assignment: "Who CARES if Shylock is treated fairly or not? He's not even REAL!"

Dick continues to feel well - with some slight shortness of breath, though he's been doing construction work at church and the shortness of breath generally follows some significant physical exercise. He is hopefully over an ear infection, which required 2 courses of antibiotics. He now is trying to reach the surgeon so he can get rid of Bob [our affectionate name for the ileostomy.]

I continue to be delighted with the lessons that I learned during Dick's illness - especially the part about how we can't change our circumstances, but we can change how we respond to them. (Mind you, I forget that lesson sometimes, like when I gave the finger to the telephone when I was irritated, irate and irrational.) I feel that I'm growing up in some areas of my life - able to be a little more confident in my dealings with parents at school, for example - but the more I work

*with the youth group, the LESS grown up I feel in other ways! I'm
content with where I am right now.*
Mom and Pop came for Thanksgiving. *J picked them up 'cause
Mary Ellen doesn't want them to drive any more for long unfamiliar
routes - good plan. They're both doing well - more forgetful, but basically
they're just growing older a little at a time.*
*We bought a little pool table - an early Christmas present - very
much fun.*
*OK. That about wraps it up. Let us know of any new specific prayer
requests for you.*
Love,
Nance

****

November 30, 1998
I called the travel agency today. In fact they did not cancel Jeremy's
plane reservations. They assured me that they could not have done
such a thing because they would have had to have his tickets to do that.
They conjectured that the airline canceled Jeremy's reservation to free
up seats and then blamed the poor defenseless travel agent. Not nice.

****

December, 1998
Each year we send out a Christmas letter to friends, many of whom
we do not see all year. I started the Christmas 1998 letter by saying that
*1998 has been the single most exciting, eventful, distressing, and
joyful year of growth in the history of the Kline family. We never could
have imagined or planned the timing of all the events that have occurred;
this has clearly been the work of the One Who knows all and loves us
completely.*
I chronicled the events of the year, and ended by saying,
*I don't think the cancer has necessarily made us appreciate each
other more - we've always done that pretty well - but it has made us look
at life a bit differently: one day at a time and with incredible gratefulness
that in the midst of trouble, God never leaves us alone. Because He
came to earth as a baby 2000 years ago, and grew up as a child,
teenager and man, He experienced all those emotions and pains that*

73

THROUGH THE BARREN TREES

we've experienced. *What a joy to know that He understands and loves us!*

Cloudburst:

January 1999 - February 1999

Chapter 10

January 18, 1999
Email from me to Ray and Jan

Things are a bit discombobulated here because Dick is back in the hospital. He got put together fine [the surgery to close the ileostomy] *on Monday the 11th and progressed very well, coming home on Wednesday. It seemed quick, but he was feeling great - eating, having diarrhea, playing pool with J (odd combination there, eh?) On Friday, he started to feel not so good - nauseous, anorexic, quite distended (no fever). By Friday night he was having a lot of pain and the dry heaves. The MD had started him on Reglan in hopes of moving things along (the diarrhea had practically stopped), but that and Compazine and Percocet failed to help (he vomited up the latter), so Jeremy and I brought him back in Friday night. That was 3 days ago, and frankly, he's not any better. However, they have found some things out. (As you know, when one is in a teaching hospital, things get done even though it is a weekend.) They took a chest X-ray, blood cultures, urine culture and stool culture and did a CAT scan. It appears that the culprit is once again C-diff, causing thickening of the colon wall (and fever - 102.6), so things just aren't going through as they should, but the CT scan did confirm that there is no obstruction. (YES!) He was quite dehydrated, so not putting much out, so they put a catheter in, which, surprise, surprise, didn't let much out! He's had an NG tube in twice - first to empty him (not much there, so they took it out) and the second time to give him the contrast dye for the CAT scan. They are on the second med now to treat the C-diff (first Flagyl, now Vancomycin), but he still is in a lot of pain (presumably gas) and he still looks 7 months pregnant.*

Poor guy. Honestly, I think this is the sickest I've seen him - not in terms of "dangerous" or life-threatening sick, but in terms of just feeling rotten. He is having diarrhea again, but even that, though good in a way, was tough because he was getting tangled in all his tubes when he would try to get up to the commode. Anyway, he said the NG tube is out again, and they are down to one IV instead of two.

Jeremy left on the train to go back to school this am. (Could we pause here for a commercial break? He got his grades, and we were all (especially J) amazed at how well he did - 3.82 [GPA] (!) I guess he takes after his father and his Aunt Jan rather than his mother. I NEVER got that high in college.) Anyway, it is encouraging to us that he really is working hard and enjoying his studies. Bad news for this semester is *that one of his classes directly conflicts with his small group Bible Study, and another class conflicts with 1/2 of his Thursday night "First Year Fellowship." I'm praying that he will really seek out fellowship somewhere. He's saying he won't come home again until May - it'll be a long 4 months - the longest he's ever been away.*

Saturday night I went sledding briefly with Zach and Olivia - terrifying, but fun. We watched Mask of Zorro - entertaining. .

How are you? Sad that it takes bad news to get me to communicate with you!

Love you both. Want to come visit soon?

Nance

****

January 18, 1999

Mom Kline is taking this present hospitalization quite hard. She is sure that the doctors have messed up somehow. She is basically angry that this is happening to her son, and she naturally would like to be able to blame someone. We talked for quite a while two nights ago; it is really hard for her to handle Dick's being ill and her not being able to do anything to help. She pointed out, quite correctly, that a mother's feelings for a child are unique and very strong. I need to remember that she is really hurting for him now and though we may not see the situation from exactly the same perspective, we can support each other.

Yesterday morning I took a walk during Sunday School class. It was a good walk, warm in the beautiful sunshine, and I spent the time just talking with God, my heavenly Father. I asked what I should be doing in response to our current problems, and the answer came in remembering one of the songs from our wedding: "Lord, make me an instrument of Thy peace", the St. Francis of Assisi prayer. I particularly thought of the part that says, "Grant that I may not so much seek to be consoled as to console; to be understood as to understand; to be loved, as to love. . . " I want that to be my prayer.

****

77

January 20, 1999

I decided to take the day off today to be with Dick, since he has developed some more problems. I went to school for about two hours until a substitute was able to relieve me. Unfortunately, I did not realize until I got to the hospital (after driving completely through two different parking garages to find a parking space) that I had brought the office and medicine cabinet keys with me! I promptly called Mary, one of the school secretaries, and she assured me that the custodian had found extra keys for my sub. What a relief!

Dick was transferred to the Step Down Unit yesterday afternoon so he could be watched more closely - on a cardiac monitor. They gave him quite a bit of Lasix yesterday, which helped him to get rid of a lot of he fluid he was holding, but also sent his potassium level plummeting. The low potassium, combined with the Demerol pain medicine, has served to make him somewhat disoriented. Last night he was seeing people in the TV - when it was off - along with his reflection. At first I thought he might be just seeing the equipment in the room and thinking it was people, but he was quite specific. He saw his mother and a few other faces he recognized, but mostly he said the people in the TV were "70's people." He seemed to know that they weren't really there, but at the same time he was surprised that I couldn't see them surrounding his bed.

When I came in today, he asked, "Is it frozen?"

"Is what frozen?" I responded.

"The turtle," he answered.

"What turtle?"

"You said you left a turtle in the Caravan."

I wonder where that came from?!

Shortly after I arrived, Dick told me that something had happened last night that he wanted to talk to me about, but not until we could talk privately. I told him there was no one else in the room (he is in a private room) but he indicated that "they sometimes listen from the next room" (pointing to the empty bathroom.) When I assured him that we were alone, he told me that in the middle of the night the staff started having a big party in the hall and there seemed to be a lot of gurneys in his room, but no one on them. He felt that his nurse was rather cruel in that she restrained him, but he wasn't being aggressive towards anyone! I reminded him that he had been restrained for his own protection because he had pulled out his nasogastric tube.

He had some apparently vivid dreams, and sometimes seemed to not completely come out of his dream world when he awoke. Sometimes he talked - about work or airplanes - with people that he apparently could see, but I could not. While he was dreaming, he would often speak or make motions. Apparently one of his dreams was a war game he and Zachary were playing in the woods near our house.

"He thinks he's the king of the world and in a few months he'll be dead," he told me.

"Who?" I asked.

"Hitler."

"Hitler? He already is dead."

"But you have to take this in relation to history. Zach."

"You mean the game you were playing with Zach in the woods?"

"Yes. I've told you that many times."

Later he whispered, "Look. There's a German soldier with a sword!"

Fortunately, some of the figures he saw went away when he reached out to touch them. Also, fortunately, he had some times today when he was completely rational and lucid, such as asking if I had called someone at work for him, and talking about going on disability since he has not been able to work.

After a long while today of Dick's sleeping, waking, and obviously seeing things that weren't there, I went down to the hospital coffee shop, where I saw Dr. Bleday. I explained that Dick was "pretty loopy" and shortly after that, the doctor came up to check on him. When Dr. Bleday walked in, Dick woke up completely and was completely alert and oriented. This made me look rather foolish, so I asked him if he still saw the people in the TV. "No," he answered.

After Dr. Bleday left, I said, "What's up? You've been saying really funny things all afternoon."

"I know I've been saying funny things," he responded.

"You mean to tell me you really didn't see any people in the television when Dr. Bleday was here?" I asked.

"Oh, I saw them all right, but I didn't want to tell him that!"

The medical folks agreed with me that Demerol was probably causing a lot of the hallucinations. Dick had a "happy button" that he could push at will for pain control, but because his fingers were a bit twitchy, I think he pushed it more than he needed too, so he was keeping the levels of Demerol as high as they could be. At least he wasn't having trouble with pain.

Dr. Bleday discontinued the Demerol, but Dick managed to have one more very vivid hallucination before the effects wore off completely. We had just had a very coherent conversation, and then Dick sat staring out into the hall, giving me a vivid description of what he saw.

"That's quite a statue out there. It's very elaborate. It moves very slowly with the wind. The little guy is putting his foot up to climb up it now and the girl is just standing in front."

I went out into the hall to the object he was describing so eloquently. It was a metal frame with a piece of canvas draped over it - a piece of equipment used for weighing people who couldn't stand on a scale. I picked up the piece of canvas to show him that it was just a piece of equipment - not a statue - and returned to the room to ask him, "Did it still look like a statue when I was touching it ?"

He was not at all pleased with me when he answered, "You've completely wrecked it and they'll probably make me pay for it!"

So much for trying to introduce reality into a drug affected mind!

****

January 22, 1999

I took the day off again to be with Dick. He is completely over the hallucinations now. Yesterday he was able to explain to me that he had had five different kinds:

1. "Virtual reality" dreams, where he had real physical involvement with a dream, but he would realize when he awoke that certain things were not there. He would drift from one world to the other (dream world to reality).

2. Hallucinations that seemed very real until he touched them, and then they would disappear.

3. Visual effects that were recognized at the time as being drug induced; for example, dots on the ceiling that looked like letters or looked as though they were moving towards him but could not be removed by touching them.

4. Visual effects that he knew were drug induced but were not touchable or explainable; for example, people in the TV along with his reflection - constant, but moving.

5. The least explainable hallucination was the one that did not disappear with touching and was present when he was awake - the "statue".

80

Dick is improving medically as well as mentally. His urine output has greatly increased so that his catheter has been removed. He is still receiving intravenous potassium and calcium because his levels of these elements are still low. He had significant trouble breathing several nights ago due to fluid in his lungs, but the lungs have been clear for the past couple of days. He has not had any fever, and his pain seems to be under control. He still has a rather large belly, but he is passing some gas and having some diarrhea. The fluid in his legs (which had made them huge) has finally started to mobilize. The big news today is that Dr. Bleday is permitting him to have a glazed donut from Dunkin' Donuts along with his clear liquids. He is going to start him on solid food tomorrow.

****

January 23, 1999
After visiting Dick yesterday, I went to Zach's wrestling match against Walpole's rival town. We lost the war, but Zach won his battle. It was an awesome match, with the score being tied at 4-4; then each of the wrestlers was ahead for a short time, until Zach pinned his opponent with only 10 seconds left in the match!

Today I had an interesting experience after driving Zachary to wrestling practice. I was making a left turn at an intersection, and the woman driving behind me bumped into my car. She was driving a minivan and had taped a block to the accelerator because she was too short to reach the pedal. Apparently it got stuck, so even though she jammed her left foot on the brake, it didn't stop the car fast enough. We were both jolted, and she was very shaken, but there seemed to be no damage to either car. However, a policeman observed the accident, so he decided to write it up, despite the lack of damage. While he was doing that, Darlene, the other woman, invited me to sit in her van with her. She was very apologetic - glad that there were no children in my car. I told her I forgave her and said that things were just a little rough for me lately since my husband was in the hospital. She replied that we all have our problems; her mom and sister were in two different hospitals - both with cancer. Her sister, the mother of a small daughter, was not expected to survive this bout with Hodgkin's Disease.

Darlene told me she would pray for my husband, and I, in uncharacteristic fashion, asked if I could pray right then for her sister and mom. She readily agreed and took my hand in both of hers. I prayed for her and her mother and sister and niece and prayed that she would know God's peace and know Him as Lord and Savior. She had tears on her cheeks when we finished; she thanked me for praying and said, "Maybe all this happened for reason." I decided that I would like to send her a copy of a book I read recently called Angel Behind the Rocking Chair. It has nothing to do with cancer or illness (it was written by a woman who had a child who was born with Down Syndrome), but I found it very uplifting. It is basically about finding oneself in a place where one did not plan to be - does not really want to be, and yet experiencing God's grace and love and joy despite the circumstances. In addition to sending Darlene the book, I am also going to try to remember to pray for her and her family.

This afternoon I talked with Dick about how quickly my perspective changes, depending on how well or poorly things around me are going. It is relatively easy now to just trust God, leaving "things" in His hands and taking one day at a time when circumstances are rough; yet when things are going well, I get caught back up in the rat race of planning and doing instead praying and trusting. I still have so much to learn!

Dick is doing well today - so well that the nurse disconnected him from both the monitor and the IV, so we were able to take walks without pushing the pole that held his equipment. It is possible that he might be discharged tomorrow, depending on whether or not his calcium level is high enough. I would like to know that solid food is definitely not bothering him before he comes home.

A couple of nights while Dick has been in the hospital I had more of those disturbing dreams that make me wake up feeling unsettled. I finally prayed in the name of Jesus that the dreams would be gone, and again they were! How encouraging!

****

February 4, 1999

Dick came home a week and a half ago after a total of ten days in the hospital. On the day he was discharged, they discovered that a blood level that has something to do with the pancreas was elevated. They were a bit concerned, but when an ultrasound showed the pancreas, gall bladder, etc. to be okay, they decided to let him go. He has been making steady progress since then - no fevers, no pain sufficient to require medication, his legs are back to their normal shape, and he has lost about 35 pounds. We had to switch sides of the bed for sleeping because he has to get up a lot at night to use the bathroom, but I'm getting used to it. It is really good to have him home! Two days after Dick came home, I had a wonderful surprise at work. I went in to find pink paper chains hanging from my office doorway - sort of like "love beads" from the 70's. It was School Nurse Appreciation Day, and that was just one of many kind recognitions of the day: plants, gifts, songs, and a multitude of wonderful cards - mostly handmade by the students. It took me days to read them all, and I have not yet been able to bring myself to recycle them. I felt so special and appreciated. It was one of my busiest days this year, but that was okay. I only wish everyone could have his or her own special day. It came at such a perfect time for me after this past year - and especially right after Dick's hospitalization. I hope people realize how much I appreciated that day.

A few days ago I mailed a copy of <u>Angel Behind the Rocking Chair</u> to Darlene. I mailed it just before 5:00 PM, and she called me the next day to thank me for it. She doesn't even live in this town, so I was amazed that she got it so fast. We talked for a while and she told me a bit more of the hardships she has endured. She understood about Dick's surgery, because she has also had bowel surgery. She has gone through some rough times but she remains upbeat and concerned about others.

Dick expects to return to work in a few days - perhaps working shortened days at first. He will continue with some medications to help with abdominal discomfort and to continue to fight the C-diff.

****

February 8, 1999

Well, here we are again - back in the emergency room. Dick called me at work at about 1:30 today to say that he had gone home around noon because of a recurrence of abdominal distension and pain. He does not have a fever, but he said it feels like the start of the C-diff that brought him to the hospital last time. We are puzzled, because he hasn't finished the Vancomycin yet, and that certainly has been working, so it doesn't <u>seem</u> as though C-diff could be the problem again, but if it is not that, then what is it? We trust that the blood work and x-ray will be able to identify the problem. It would be nice if it was a simple problem and he could go home.

I am really not ready for another crisis. I am of the opinion that crises should come one at a time, yet we view one of Jeremy's recent decisions as a crisis, and Zach is also facing a conflict. Jeremy just decided to join a fraternity. This came as a big surprise to us, because we had not thought that he would be interested. He called us last Friday night to talk about the financial aspects of joining a fraternity, and I, in my typically undiplomatic manner, proceeded to list the reasons why I thought that fraternities were bad (social cliques, drinking, etc.). Dick on the other hand, in his own quiet way that encourages the listener to really listen, simply challenged Jeremy to "pursue God." Jeremy seemed to really ponder what Dick was saying, so we were quite surprised that he made the final decision to join the fraternity that a couple of his friends were also joining. I feel a bit more relaxed about the whole thing now because I wrote Jeremy a letter outlining my concerns, but ending the letter quite positively. I had both Dick and Zach read it and I reread it to make sure it sounded okay before mailing it .

Zach's crisis is probably as upsetting to me as it is to him. We just found out that Olivia's prom (she does not go to the same high school as Zach) is on the same night as his high school pops concert, and since band is one of his school subjects, he is required to attend this performance as part of his grade.

I'd like to resolve one crisis before moving on to the next! Control: that is what I like, but I do not have it. I have to wait. Meanwhile, the one thing over which I have any control is my attitude. I was a bit shaky when Dick called earlier today to say that he had to go back to the hospital, but I'm better now.

****

February 27,1999

The doctors identified Dick's problem as adhesions, and although these can reportedly reoccur at any time, this episode resolved spontaneously, and he has had no recurrence up to this point. So the medical situation is stable, and family life continues.

I talked to my friend Anne a week ago, and she gave me a wonderful analogy with regard to parenting adolescents. Here's the story: When deer reach adolescence, they need to rub the fur off their antlers, and the way they do that is to go up to a tree and rub the antlers against the tree. We as parents need to be the "trees" for our children as they "rub their antlers" in an effort to work out the issues they face as they grow. It is important that we stand firm so we'll be there for them. We shouldn't go after them (trees don't move), nor should we back off and "flex" in our convictions (trees don't move.) Their rubbing may injure our bark a little, but it won't kill us, and if we are there for them, they will keep coming back when more "fur" needs to be rubbed off - when they have more questions or issues to discuss.

I found that analogy helpful.

Mostly Sunny:

March 1999 - June 1999

Chapter 11

April 10, 1999
Email from Dick to several of our friends
Thanks one and all for your many prayers.

As many of you know, I had some reconstructive surgery (ileostomy takedown) in January, which went very well except for a third, and worse yet, bout with the C-Diff infection which followed 5 days later, landing me in the hospital for yet another 10 days. However, since then I am happy to report that my health has continued to improve weekly to the point where I am almost back to normal. I'm feeling well enough that I am actually going on a trip for work one week from now. This is something I wouldn't even have considered 5 or 6 weeks ago. Please pray that I will always find a bathroom close by when I - often urgently - need one :-) Haven't been well enough for over a year to even consider such a thing. Praise God!

A couple of weeks ago I had an appointment with my oncologist. This was the first four month check up after the completion of my chemotherapy. I'll continue to have regular four month check ups for some time to come.

I just received a letter from my oncologist summarizing the results. I found the news good enough to share it with you all.

"Dear Mr. Kline:
I just wanted to let you know that your laboratory work from 3/22/99 was all fine. Your white count was a little on the low side, but nothing of concern. This is certainly consistent with the course of treatment you had. Everything else looks great.
Please give me a call should you have any questions or concerns."

I'll add that everything feels great (most of the time) as well! Praise God, and thanks for your many prayers; they certainly have been answered.

God bless you all,
Dick

****

June 1, 1999

May 21 was Olivia's prom and Zach's pops concert. The way the conflict was finally resolved was that Zach fulfilled his responsibility to the band and Olivia went to her prom - with Jeremy! It seemed the perfect solution; Jeremy was home from college, and had gotten a tux for Christmas, so we figured that we would not have to worry about that expense. I paid for the flowers, and since it was "all in the family", Zach could go out with Olivia after the prom and concert. As it turned out, it was a bit more expensive than expected, since Jeremy forgot to bring his tux home from school! By the time he went to rent one, there were no more great "deals", but at least he didn't get stuck with some weird color like lime green! Before the concert and prom, we took pictures of Olivia with both the boys; Zach was dressed in black pants, white shirt and bow tie for the concert, so the boys just had to share the jacket for the pictures. Dick and I went to the concert, and I believe the evening was pleasant for everyone.

Last weekend we took a mini vacation to the Roaring Brook Ranch and Tennis Resort in the Adirondack Mountains in New York. I had been looking for a place that was in reasonable driving distance that would offer a measure of entertainment for all of us. It was actually quite enjoyable. Even though it was a holiday weekend (Memorial Day) it was not exceptionally crowded. The "resort" aspect meant that a lot was included in the price we paid: breakfasts, dinners, tennis lessons and trail rides on the horses.

After the first ride - at the "medium" level, we decided to go up a level for our second ride. The boys had both had riding lessons several years ago, and Dick and I had each ridden a little at different times in the past, so we thought we could handle a little faster action than the first ride. All went well until we started galloping. I rounded a corner on my horse just in time to see Dick roll over on the ground and get up to run after his horse, which had just thrown him! I was completely amazed at the grace with which he executed that fall and roll; no doubt it was his high school judo experience that taught him the fine art of falling! That afternoon we both decided, at the boys' urging - and since it was our twenty-third anniversary weekend - to splurge for one of the few things that wasn't included in the daily cost: massages.

Lightening Strikes Again:

July 1999

Chapter 12

July 9, 1999

I am currently at New England Frontier Camp in Maine, once again volunteering as camp nurse for the week. I finally have a little time to catch up on my journaling.

Jeremy did extremely well academically for his first year at UVA, ending with a grade point average over 3.8. He loves school and is looking forward to returning. He is once again spending the summer as a life guard at Camp Berea, even though his friend Pete was not able to return with him. So far he seems to be doing well there. Before he left for camp, he agreed to paint the front of the house for us to pay back his debt incurred by overspending his "allowance" at school. This, incidentally, involved a great example of Dick's wisdom in dealing with Jeremy. While I would have been inclined to press for details on how he spent his money and proceed to correct him in his errors in judgment, Dick simply pointed out to him that the money was not his to spend. This far better approach allowed Jeremy to think it through and willingly take responsibility for paying back the money.

Zach has also been doing well. He just (barely) got his license after six months of mother terror as he practiced driving - yet another area in which Dad greatly excelled in parenting; he's a much better, much less anxious driving teacher. Zach continues to be strongly committed to God and our church youth group. He is still dating Olivia, and although they spend a great deal of time being together or talking on the phone, she did not apparently object to his decision to spend the summer at New England Frontier Camp.

Life for me has been bordering on hectic with the end of school and concern for my parents. It has been clear that they are going to need some assistance, as Mom is forgetting more and having difficulty with anything but the simplest of meal preparations. The original thought was for my sister Mary Ellen and her husband Phil to move back from Michigan to Auburn, Massachusetts, where they used to live and my parents still live. They intended to purchase a home with an in-law apartment. Phil does not have a job in this area, but he could probably leave his current job in March, 2000; however, Mary Ellen feels a real urgency to be with our parents sooner. Their daughter Becky has meanwhile moved in with her grandparents, but this is at best a temporary solution. However, it certainly has been wonderful to know that they are not alone, and it is good for Becky to have a place to live while looking for a job.

We had a family meeting with Dick and me, Mary Ellen and Phil, and Dan and Marcia Curtis (Mom and Dad's pastor and his wife, who are also good friends of theirs.) The idea was to "brainstorm" other options with Mom and Dad since Mary Ellen and Phil were unable to find a suitable house with an in-law apartment. I had already researched assisted living places, and I presented several to them, saving the best for last: The Woods at Eddy Pond, which is in Auburn. Mom and Dad were both surprisingly open to the idea of moving to an assisted living facility. It was a bit difficult for Mom, thinking of leaving her home of almost 50 years, but Dad was practically ready to move in before we got out of the car when we later went to visit it. Mary Ellen and Phil subsequently found a house (without an in-law apartment) and plan to move in early September.

All seemed to be moving along very well, except that Mom and Dad were just on the waiting list for The Woods and all the people in the one bedroom apartments were currently healthy and happy. I really couldn't imagine how God could work this all out. I had hoped that Mom and Dad could move during the summer, while I was off from school and therefore more available, but there just seemed to be no way. I was therefore pleasantly surprised when the marketing director at The Woods mentioned The Lodge at Eddy Pond, a facility right next door. It has the same architecture and all the amenities (meals three times a day, security, transportation, etc.) except personal care, but with slightly bigger apartments and lower cost. The big plus is the current availability of a choice of apartments. There are even a few incentives, such as a $500 moving allowance and one month free rent! I told Dad about this place on a Thursday night at 7:00, and by 9:00 he had already visited it! He had made a deposit by the next day, and soon after that we set up a moving date for July 27. Here was a classic example of God being able to do "immeasurably more than all we ask or imagine." (Ephesians 3:20)

Having plans for my parents in place, it was with some sense of peace that I came up here to camp on Thursday, July 1, after accompanying Dick for a colonoscopy. Dr. Bleday had intended to do a "follow-up" colonoscopy a year after Dick's initial surgery for cancer, but it was delayed because of all his complications. Dr. Bleday told us on Thursday that he found a little something - a little ulcer-like thing - up higher in the colon than where Dick had received radiation. He said it did not look like cancer, but he biopsied it and said he would call with the pathology report in a day or two. Dick had heard nothing when he came up to visit Zach and me last Saturday, July 3, so he called Dr. Bleday on Sunday when he got home.

Dick called me Sunday night to say that the cancer is back. I hung up the phone and sobbed on Bobbie's shoulder. She had been here for the previous week and had hoped to leave for home early on Monday morning, but she delayed her departure to make sure that I was okay. As Camp Health Services Director, she tried to get a replacement for me so that I could go home early, but it did not work out. I am sorry to not be with Dick now (he had a CAT scan yesterday and was to meet with Dr. Bleday this morning) but I guess this is where I am supposed to be this week.

I think I could rank Tuesday, July 6, as one of the worst days of my life. I went to bed Monday night with the knowledge that my husband has a recurrence of cancer 16 months following his original diagnosis. Intellectually, I can recognize that the odds are not good, although I am really not ready or willing to fully accept that. God can choose to heal him again - and without complications - if He wants. Nonetheless, it is not a particularly happy thought to consider surgery, hospitalization, and maybe more chemo or radiation.

I managed to finally get to sleep with those thoughts running through my mind, only to be wakened before 2:00 AM with the news that an eleven year old diabetic camper was not responding, and the counselors were unable to get frosting in him to combat the probable insulin reaction. I wonder if I will ever forget that terror: throwing on a jumpsuit over my nightgown; grabbing my glasses; running to the health office to snatch the nurse's trauma bag as well as glucose (sugar) paste and Glucagon (sugar injection); and jumping in the camp station wagon with the other "in charge" people to hopefully go make everything better! Because David was a younger camper, his cabin was in the Stockade area, which is located about one third to one half mile away from the main camp. The person who had come down to the main camp to alert us was not a driver, so he had run the entire distance to awaken us, there being no phones or radio system to alert us.

David was located upstairs in the most distant of the Stockade cabins. His friend Carl had awakened and called David's name with no response. Their counselor awakened to find David breathing shallowly and gulping. By the time I arrived, the counselors had gotten some frosting on his lips and a little inside his mouth (and a lot on his pillow case) but he was still unresponsive. After fifteen more minutes of my attempting to give him glucose paste with no response (other than movement when I put my finger in his mouth), and attempting unsuccessfully to get a blood glucose reading, I told the camp director to call 911 and I gave David the Glucagon injection. That stuff was remarkable! Within five minutes, he was able to check his own glucose level, which had risen nicely. After another thirty-five minutes, the rescue squad arrived, but by this time they were not needed.

We drove David, Carl and one of their counselors back to the health lodge for David to get a snack and for them all to sleep for the remainder of the night. They slept. I, on the other hand, had a rare attack of insomnia. It wasn't until it started to get light outside - around 5:00 AM - that I finally drifted off to sleep for nearly two hours. I awoke feeling like King Darius in the Bible, running to the lions' den to see Daniel: to see if Daniel's God had spared his life. Both Daniel and David made it, but it has been a somewhat anxious week, with late night snacks and blood sugar checks and lots of prayer for David, so that we might avoid another insulin reaction.

Later on Tuesday, the day after the night of terror, thinking things could not be much worse, I got an email that Dick had forwarded from Ray and Jan. Both Ray and Jan had had routine HIV testing because of the nature of their work as doctors in Africa, where AIDS is common, and Jan's test came out positive - twice. This particular test is known to have false positives, so she was to be retested the next day with a more accurate test. We don't know any results yet.

I have not had much free time this week - no time to mope, but not much time to read or pray, either. I did have a couple of good walks and talks with Amy, the brand new wife of one of the staff members here. It was a gift, really. She is a student nurse - only one semester left - so we were able to discuss nursing issues and she helped with first aid. Even though she is young (twenty-three) she has already dealt with a lot in her life, and she was sufficiently mature to really be a friend this past week. She has gone now, but I am grateful for the time she was here.

****

July 12, 1999

I finished my time at NEFC two days ago, and Dick and I went up to Berea today to see Jeremy. We had a wonderful day, packing quite a lot into the time we had together. As a lifeguard, Jeremy had access to a speed boat and water skiing equipment so Dick skied (slalom), Jeremy did wake boarding, and I spent considerable time in the water, failing in my attempts to ski. I was more successful in our mountain climbing venture. We climbed Bear Mountain, which is just across the road from camp. It is not a very high mountain, but if the trail had been any steeper, or my legs any shorter, I might not have been able to move from one rock to the next in certain parts. The view of Newfound Lake from the top definitely made the effort worthwhile. I was really glad that we could have the time with Jeremy before Dick undergoes yet another surgery.

****

July 24, 1999
Dick's surgery was yesterday - in a different hospital this time, because Dr. Bleday had switched hospitals, and we felt that it was more important to stick with a doctor who knew Dick "inside out" quite literally, rather than staying with the same hospital.

Before the surgery, Dr. Bleday had presented us with three different ways that the surgery might be done, depending on what he found when he got inside. The third option - for a permanent colostomy - was immediately rejected by Dick. I had actually wanted him to do that - thinking that it would be the least complicated procedure, and he would have just as good a prognosis for "normalcy" as he was having currently, with his frequent bathroom trips and occasional incontinence. However, he said that when he had the ileostomy that he just didn't feel like himself, so he wanted to avoid the permanent colostomy if at all possible. It does seem as though he has had more bowel control in the past couple of weeks, and he expects it to eventually get even better, despite this interlude, so I finally supported him in his decision to reject the permanent colostomy.

Ray and Jan are back in the States to get Elizabeth settled at Boston University and to do some other visiting as well. Yesterday was orientation at BU, and Jan was kind enough to come from there to the hospital to wait with me during Dick's surgery. We had to wait several hours while he was in surgery, but she has an even longer wait to know about her HIV status. The Western Blot test (more sensitive than the original two she had) was "indeterminate" in Nairobi. She will have that repeated as well as some more confirming tests next week in Tennessee. It is a very difficult time for her - not knowing whether or not

94

she has a fatal disease. She is aware that a positive HIV status would not only effect her life expectancy, but also the quality of her remaining life. Would she be able to continue working as a physician in Africa or elsewhere? The medications for HIV are also quite costly, which could cause some financial strain as Liz is starting college. With all that Jan is facing, I especially appreciated that she would come to wait with me.

Dr. Bleday came down to talk to us following the surgery, which lasted about four hours. He did not have to do the more complicated procedure that he had anticipated, but because the lower part of the colon had been irradiated, the first sutures the doctors put in just came out, so they used a "different technique", successfully that time. They also did another temporary ileostomy to allow the surgical site to heal. Dr. Bleday said that this time, they will use Vancomycin prophylactically to hopefully avoid C-diff complications. He spent quite a while talking to Jan and me; he was really very kind. He admitted that the prophylaxis for C-diff is essentially uncharted territory. They will probably give Dick medication both by mouth and into the lower part of the colon, through one of the openings of the ostomy. Dick is also getting two other antibiotics and Flagyl by IV. We hope that there will be no complications of any kind this time!

My poor husband had considerable pain when he got to the recovery room last night, but with a position change and more medication, he felt a little better.   I visited him briefly, but the nurse thought it best that I return home and call from there to check on him. The second time I called, I learned he had been transferred to a private room, so I was able to talk with him there.

This morning we stopped to see Dick on the way to the airport. Ray, Jan, Elizabeth and Tim are headed to Tennessee for two weeks. Dick was in great shape. He had already been up walking and his pain was well controlled. The only trouble was that he was itchy from the medication he had gotten via his epidural catheter (left in near the spine following his receiving his anesthesia for the surgery.) They gave him something to combat the itch, but it unfortunately also combated the analgesic effects of the pain medication.   When I visited him again on the way back from the airport, he was in a great deal of pain, including feeling as though there was a tack in his back at the site of the epidural catheter. The doctors and nurses basically said, "Sorry; we'll just use lotion for the itch next time; you'll feel better soon." A few hours later he was feeling much better - and quite affectionate towards me!

****

July 25, 1999

When I called this morning, Dick wasn't feeling very well; his oxygen saturation level was down and his temperature was up, but there was nothing too bad or concrete to report. I debated whether or not I should go to church, but he promised me he would tell me if he really needed me to visit, and he said it wasn't necessary at that point. I still felt a bit torn on my way to church, but decided that I had to take my own advice and <u>choose</u> not to worry - or at least to prioritize my worries! These worries (slight fever and low oxygen saturation) were not concrete and serious enough to make it to the top of the worry list, so I decided, <u>somewhat</u> successfully, to put them aside.

Church was good; the theme was prayer, and the first scripture passage was <u>mine</u>: 1 Thessalonians 5:16-18 (Be joyful always; pray continually; give thanks in all circumstances. . .) The pastor's powerful illustration pointed out to me again that God knows best, even when things look bleak to us. Illustration: There was a man stranded on an island, waiting for rescue. He had built a hut, where he kept all his possessions. One day he took a walk across the island, and retuned to find his hut burned to the ground. He was extremely upset and angry and began to curse God. The next day, a ship came and rescued him. He asked the captain how he knew to come to the island, and the captain replied, "I came because I saw your smoke signals."

The picture often looks different from another angle.

After lunch with some church friends, I went in to the hospital to see Dick. Today's visit was much different from yesterday's two visits, since he slept much of the time, and when he was awake, he was feeling nauseous and generally lousy. I prayed for his nausea, and I prayed with much thankfulness for who he is and for the years we have had together. Though we still have not been married for more than half my life, I have known him for more years than there were before I met him. What a wonderful man - such a gift from God to me.

****

July 26, 1999

Today was the loneliest I can remember feeling. I had spoken to Dick, who said that the nasogastric tube they had put in, intending to leave it in for 45 min, was still in long after they planned to take it out.

Apparently his stomach didn't "wake up" as soon as his small intestines, so "stuff" was collecting there, creating pressure on his lungs and resulting in less than optimum breathing. I couldn't understand why God didn't answer my prayer about "no complications"; I miss Dick; Jeremy and Zach are away; our friends Arlene and Paul are away; and our next door neighbors Bob and Debbie are away. So I felt sorry for myself, but it was short lived.

****

July 31, 1999

When I last wrote, Dick was not feeling well and sleeping a lot in the hospital, but as he slept less, we talked more, or lay on the bed together resting or watching TV. It was nice that he was in a private room. The doctors and nurses would come in and make some comment about how "cute" it was for us to be on the bed together and how I shouldn't move because I was good medicine: some pleasant moments.

There were also some less than pleasant moments. One resident (physician) was personable, but a bit all-knowing and unwilling to ask for help from the lesser beings such as nurses or patient and wife. Consequently, one of Dick's procedures - inserting Vancomycin into the lower part of the colon - was not done one day because he couldn't find the hole and never bothered to come back with help! Anyway, he sort of redeemed himself the next day before Dick's discharge by coming in specifically to show me where to insert the catheter for the medicine. I've been doing this once a day at home without any difficulty.

Dick came home Wednesday afternoon, July 28. He had a lot of trouble with pain the first night, but it has gotten better, especially since he had the staples removed from his incision yesterday. Yesterday we also got the pathology report: the lymph nodes outside the colon were 1+ positive - i.e., the ones closest to the colon are malignant, but not the ones farther away from the colon. This means Dick will need chemo again, a rather disturbing thought. It is hard to understand why he has to go through so much. Why aren't our fervent prayers being answered? So many people are praying for us. Last night we also got the news that Jan's tests were <u>negative</u> - no HIV! We're <u>so</u> grateful for this - and thrilled for Ray and Jan - but why was <u>our</u> news not so good?

Dick and I think these things; we talk about them. We actually haven't cried about them this time, and I haven't even cried alone since my pity party at the beginning of the week. However, we do go back to remembering that Father knows best, and we think of the hut that burned down. None of it makes sense to us now, but maybe someday it will.

Mostly now we are enjoying each other and some rest. We watch videos and we went out for a movie matinee this afternoon, to be in an air-conditioned place. Things are quiet here right now, but there is a lot of busyness around us. Mom and Dad moved Tuesday and are quite happy, though not 100% settled. Ray, Jan, Liz and Tim are in Tennessee - due back here Tuesday, August 6. Jeremy is getting a bit worn down at camp. Zach had a few rough weeks at his camp, but is hopeful that this next one will be better. Becky started a new job. Don (Mary Ellen and Phil's son) and Maggie and their son - little Ray - are coming out here from California on August 14, and our family reunion is scheduled for August 17. Jeremy is due to go back to school August 25, probably the day after he comes home from camp. The yard sale for Mom and Dad's houseful of belongings is August 26. Meanwhile, Dick is off work, recovering at home for much of this time. The next question - hopefully to be answered somewhat after he sees Dr. Huberman on Monday - is what he should do regarding work. He is wondering about long term disability since he will have six months of chemo and another surgery and recovery. Until we figure that out, we are just going to take one day at a time.

Steady Rain:

August 1999 - December 1999

Chapter 13

August 16, 1999

One day at a time. It gets old. Yesterday was not such a good one. Nor today. Actually, Saturday wasn't that great either. Saturday Dick and I left at around 10:00AM to get Zach at NEFC in Maine. We did manage to get him all packed up before the torrential downpours. Zach drove as far as Berea in New Hampshire, where we had to trade cars with Jeremy, who had sprained his ankle a week earlier. It might have improved, had he not had the crutch give way two days earlier when he was in a department store. The x-ray at that point showed no fracture, but despite Jeremy's being on crutches with a half cast, the ankle didn't improve much, so he decided to come home for Saturday night and Sunday. Since the injury was to Jeremy's left foot, we figured he would be okay driving an automatic car, but it might be tricky for him to drive his car with standard transmission because of the clutch. We couldn't just drive him home since he had to drive back on Sunday, so we left him the Caravan, and Dick and Zach and I continued home in the little Escort.

We had supper at a Friendly's restaurant, and then an hour or so later, in the middle of listening to a mystery book on the car's tape deck, with Zach driving in the pouring rain, Dick had an accident with the ileostomy bag. There was major leakage with no clean-up supplies, since this was not the car we had originally been driving. Fortunately, there was a rest area just ahead, so we stopped there and Zach and I went in for paper towels, only to find a "towel-free" restroom environment! I grabbed toilet paper and got paper towels from a restroom maintenance person, but Zach was more creative: he emptied the baby changing station of wipes! Thankfully, he had clothes from his recent stay at camp for Dick to wear, so we were able to proceed a bit more comfortably, getting home considerably after Jeremy, who was actually worried about us. (I think it gave him a hint of what it feels like to be the parent of a teenager!)

Sunday started out fine. Dick and Zach and I went to church, but midway through the service Dick started to have back and abdominal pain. He rested a bit at home before and after lunch and decided he could go with the family out to Auburn for a gathering of family and some friends at my parents' old house. While there, he started feeling really poorly. Ray examined him a little and decided that medical intervention

100

was in order. I was going to drive him to the hospital by myself after talking with Dr. Bleday, but then he started retching, and I wasn't keen on going all the way into Boston alone with his being really sick, so Jan came with me. Meanwhile, Jeremy and Zach were headed off to see their grandparents' new place and then go together up to Berea for a couple of days before returning for the official family reunion at our house on Tuesday, the seventeenth. By this time, Maggie was also feeling quite ill. She had been sick for two days, since arriving from California, and had visited the emergency room the night before due to dehydration.

Dick felt a little better in the car, but by the time we got to the hospital, he was very uncomfortable and the back pain had gotten worse. Two doses of IV morphine did not help, and he was also given IV medications for nausea. They doctors did x-rays and blood work and inserted a nasogastric tube. The ostomy basically stopped working, though it had worked a little earlier in the day. The x-ray showed an ileus (intestinal obstruction), but they couldn't determine the cause. His pancreatic enzymes were not elevated, so they ruled out pancreatitis. Meanwhile, the darn pain was nearly driving him crazy. I finally <u>begged</u> God to give him relief; I was a bit frustrated with God at the time. Within five to ten minutes or so, he finally fell asleep and later the pain ceased completely. The doctor wondered which had given him relief: the morphine, the antinausea medication or the NG tube. I don't know which of those things He used, but I know Who got rid of Dick's pain!

This morning Jeremy called to say that he decided to end his summer at Berea today. The combination of only being able to hobble around on his crutches because of his ankle and being far away from his dad when things are not going well is a bit much, so he has decided to forego the $150 bonus for completing his contract and call it quits. I was able to make an appointment so that Jeremy was able to see his doctor about his ankle shortly after he arrived home. The report was that the ankle looks pretty bad: maybe torn ligaments, and surgery might be needed. He is to see a specialist tomorrow. Enough already.

Is it too much to ask to just have a family reunion? I had been thinking that the theme could be "Great is Thy Faithfulness" (Dick's favorite song), and I was looking forward to taking a picture of the whole family - for the first time with Maggie and little Ray. It doesn't seem that Dick will even be able to be there. Jan said this morning that maybe his absence just means we will have another time together soon; all I could think was to wonder if the next time we will all be together will be at

Dick's funeral! It is getting difficult again to view my glass as being half full.

Usually when I have visited Dick, I have felt as though I could be a comfort to him or at least that we are in this thing together. Today I felt separated because he could hardly talk with his throat pain - and I could hardly talk because of crying. I sat on his bed and didn't even want to move. (Big plus: he had the bed by the window, so I could look outside.) He hugged me a couple of times, but it was hard with his NG tube, which hurt if I hit it the wrong way. Sigh. I guess in my little pity party, I forgot that some people have it much worse. We recently listened to Christopher Reeve's autobiography on audiotape. After being paralyzed from being thrown from his horse, he had far more tubes than Dick and he couldn't move at all (still can't) but he and his wife have stuck together and moved on.

I was just thinking about that hut that burned down (the sermon illustration.) I have been reflecting on that story - how that bad incident turned out for good - but I feel as though I'm in the night after the hut burned down: at this point I have no hint that a rescue is coming and it seems like a very long night and I'm really sick of this island!!!!!!!!!!!!!!!

After sitting still ("Be still and know that I am God"), I realize that there are good things on the island: flowers, birds and fruit, and a little fresh water stream. Some of the fruit is hard to get: the berries are near thorn bushes; my knife was wrecked in the fire, so it is hard to cut the pineapples; and sometimes the monkeys get to the bananas before I do. But there is fruit and there are flowers and birds and that stream. I'd like to go sit by that stream (when it's not buggy) on a rock when the sun is shining through the trees. Maybe tomorrow...

****

August 17, 1999

Reunion Day. Months in the planning, but it just wasn't complete, with Dick still in the hospital and Maggie still sick. This frustrated and angered me. When one is already distressed, little irritations can be intolerable. Such was the case today. I woke up a half hour late this morning - with a headache. · I slipped in water leaking from the refrigerator and later found a puddle in front of the dryer and thought the washer was leaking also (not so; it was just water from a wet shirt). Jan was <u>wonderful</u> with taking over the food preparation for this reunion - even buying and preparing my dishes my way, which I am sure was not easy for her. I really tried to let go of things, but I kept butting in while she was working in the kitchen - unable to relinquish control of how my recipes were prepared.

I decided to go with Jeremy's to his doctor's appointment about his ankle, but he left before me, since he was getting x-rays first. By the time I was ready to leave, it seemed that the entire Walpole Department of Public Works with half of their equipment had gathered in front of our house. When I made a motion that I needed to get the car out of the driveway, they all shook their heads to indicate that this would not be possible. I motioned again (since speech was not possible over the sound of the jackhammer that was digging up the road) that I really needed to get out, and Mr. Jackhammer pointed to Mr. Big Guy, who came over to me, again shaking his head, "No." I said that I really needed to get out, and he asked why. ("None of his business!" I thought.) I told him it was for a doctor's appointment, and he decided that he might be able to back up his truck a bit so I could squeeze by. (I successfully avoided the workers' toe and shovels, but was unable to avoid the loose tar. Sigh.)

Halfway down the next street, I realized I had not brought along a book to read while waiting at the doctor's office. Scream. Really.

I felt particularly angry because of these minor irritations on top of my major frustrations and concluded that if I was stopped for speeding, I would simply cry quietly and then ask the police officer before he left if I could borrow his gun. Hmmm.

Jeremy's appointment went better than expected. It does not appear that either surgery or even extensive rehabilitation will be needed for his ankle as was originally thought. The rehab doctor agreed (with consult to an orthopedic doctor) that the ankle is not broken, but tendons and ligaments are injured and will need time to heal. This doctor gave specific directions to Jeremy about increasing activity and exercise for that ankle and gradually increasing weight bearing. Bicycling and swimming will be okay, but it appears that tennis will not be an option this semester.

Dick's NG tube was removed today. That was a good thing, in the midst of multiple frustrations.

****

August 22, 1999

After gradually increasing Dick's intake and making sure that he did not have pain after eating, the doctors finally discharged him on Friday, August 20. Jeremy picked him up. He started to feel quite well after he got home, but he remained tired.

Meanwhile, we had reserved and paid most of the cost for renting a truck on Wednesday, the eighteenth, to bring some of our things out to Auburn for a yard sale at my parents' home. The plan was to take some of their things, such as their dining room table and lawn mower, and sell ours instead. We also planned to pick up my dad's antique grandfather clock. I was not too excited about driving the 14 foot rental truck, but Ray said he had driven more difficult vehicles in more difficult circumstances in Africa, so he didn't mind driving. I was very happy about that!

Zach helped us load it up; he has Dick's sense about the right way to do that sort of thing. Ray and I then headed off to Auburn, where Phil and his sister and mother and my parents were waiting. Phil was most helpful in unloading our things, and his sister Leslie was incredibly helpful in loading the truck back up with the things my parents were giving us. I had brought some ropes - but not enough - and a roll of packing tape, intending to put a box together. Leslie managed to use the packing tape instead of ropes, so we were able to transport the dining room table, several small chairs, two stuffed chairs, a sleeper sofa, the lawn mower, the snow blower and the priceless, precious grandfather clock completely unharmed. Les was also full of hints - about lawn maintenance and general life tips such as: "Always keep a roll of duct tape in your car."

****

September 1, 1999

Although Dick continued to feel reasonably well after coming home from the hospital, he was still quite tired, so it was decided that Jan would drive down to UVA with Jeremy and me, and we would leave Dick at home for R & R. We left Walpole at about 10:30 PM last Tuesday, August 24, and arrived in Charlottesville around 9:30 AM on Wednesday, the twenty-fifth. Jeremy drove the entire way with just pit stops for gas and one unplanned stop in Connecticut at around 12:30 AM, when a trailer truck drove by us, with the driver madly honking his horn and pointing at the roof of our van. We pulled off at the next exit to find that the box carrier on top of the van had opened, because the rear latch had broken off. We would have had no means to secure it closed, except that at the last minute before leaving home, I went to make a final check of Jeremy's room. I noticed a roll of duct tape on the floor, so I picked it up and threw it in the car, remembering Leslie's directive. Duct tape is just the ticket for closing a car top box! We had no further problems, except one wrong choice of route around Washington D.C. at the beginning of rush hour, which delayed us a little.

When we arrived at Jeremy's fraternity house, no one was up, so Jan and I carried a lot of his things up to his room on the third floor; Jeremy was still unable to walk well on his bad ankle. Jan and I were amazed at the state of the building - very odiferous and full of trash! Jeremy informed us that the dumpster had not been emptied all summer, and that was why the trash was still in the house. The windows were all open - presumably because of the smell - so the mosquitoes entered freely and feasted on us as we labored up the stairs. Jeremy's room was not as bad as some of the other rooms. The fellow who had lived in the room last year had cleaned it up nicely. There was no mattress, but there was a good amount of built in storage space. The bathroom light and one of the faucets didn't work, and the door was off one of the showers. When Jeremy asked me, "What do you think, Mom?" I managed to answer truthfully that "it has potential and I like the built-ins."

Unfortunately, my best efforts to not cry failed when it was time to say good-bye. It wasn't as bad as last year, but for several miles after we left, I couldn't really speak to Jan. I think it was hard leaving him in the fraternity house with no mom or dorm counselor to help - especially when he had a bum leg and so much work to do.

Jan and I arrived back here on Thursday. It was quite pleasant traveling with Jan - good conversation, which greatly helped to pass the time. She and Tim left for Nairobi on Sunday, while Ray stayed to help get Liz settled at BU.

Monday was Dick's first day of the new round of chemotherapy - this time he is getting CPT-11. I went to the hospital with him, since we didn't really know what the immediate effects would be. We had been told that the most likely side effect, if any, would be diarrhea. That might be a bit difficult to monitor because of the ileostomy, which produces loose stool normally. While we were waiting for him to get started, Dick read the information about this particular chemo drug. It was a bit disheartening, because the studies that have been done of CPT-11, on patients with advanced adenocarcinoma, showed that it has been

105

effective in one out of seven patients in reducing the size of tumors which could not be treated surgically and which were unresponsive to 5-FU (the first chemotherapy drug that Dick had.) He wonders if it is worth the trouble, but the fact is that there have not been studies done on people in his situation - those with a second primary cancer site. Maybe the 5-FU (the first chemotherapy drug) was partially effective on this second tumor (and that's why it looked atypical to Dr. Bleday) and maybe the CPT-11 is actually more effective at this level than on advanced tumors. I do think that there is some mind-body connection, and that we should assume that this chemo will help him.

As Dick was receiving the chemo on Monday, he experienced some cramping in his lower colon, so they gave him some medication for that (atropine). Then he had cramps in his upper intestines, so they gave him another drug (Imodium). That effectively stopped the cramping, but also slowed up his digestive tract for the next 48 hours! Because of his history, we were a little concerned about an ileus. Also, he had a headache until Tuesday night. It could have been either from the anti-nausea med he had before the chemo or from the chemo itself. We just hope the next time is better!

****

September 27, 1999

Sunday before last was the Eighteenth Annual House Church Reunion. As usual, it was here at our house, and as always, it was wonderful to gather with these people who have stayed connected with us since the mid seventies. This reunion had two especially bright spots: one was an outstanding Anne Hulley chocolate cake to celebrate three birthdays (Dick, Barb and Charlie) and the other was a time of singing and prayer to celebrate God's faithfulness. To "help" with the singing, as we sang I "unscrolled" a banner that Anne had made of the entire song "Great is Thy Faithfulness". She had sent it to us several months ago - said she had worked on it a little at a time over a period of several weeks. It is about seven inches high and over one hundred feet long. I think Dick found it a bit distracting that I unrolled it during the singing, but I felt that it was a real work of art and should be appreciated by more than just us two!

Chapter 14

October 3, 1999
Email from me to Jan
Dear JAN (and Ray),
Thanks for your news filled and thoughtful and encouraging letter.
Last weekend I went to a women's retreat at Berea where the theme was something like "Weaving a Fabric of Faith." It was clear that the theme would include such things as going through hard times in one's life, and I had these visions of sharing that my husband had cancer and people feeling sorry for me and encouraging me and maybe even learning something specific about dealing with cancer, blah, blah, blah. Well, none of the above happened - it was clear that EVERYBODY has tough things in their lives, but those things weren't talked about much. The speaker was quite good, but the first thing that really grabbed me was when these two women - the Morgan Sisters - came Saturday night to sing. They sang music that was of a style that doesn't generally particularly excite me - mostly basic hymns, and they weren't at all showy, but the message came across loud and clear. They sang "How Great Thou Art" and - big surprise - I got a sense of how GREAT God is. Then they sang a song about the greatest battle of all time and how the cross stood on the line between the opposing forces, and when Jesus died and said "It is finished," that was the END of the war; when Jesus died, he took care of everything. There are still skirmishes, but the war is over. Jesus won, and that's the bottom line from which we can face all of life's little and big problems.
Such a simple message. We KNEW it when we accepted Him, but we still need reminders. I'm grateful He is still willing to give them - in many forms in ways we are each able to hear them.
Another thing I got from the weekend was the motivation to memorize Lamentations 3: 19-?. I'm sure I heard it before and actually knew a lot of the second part, but going back to verse 19 explains how the writer gets to the latter part. You don't have to look it up, 'cause I'd like to quote it for you. It took me several days to be able to say it this smoothly: "I remember my affliction and my wandering, the bitterness and the gall. I well remember them, and my soul is downcast within me. Yet this I call to mind, and therefore I have hope: Because of the Lord's great love, we are not consumed. His compassions never fail; they are

107

new every morning. Great is your faithfulness. I say to myself, 'The Lord is my portion; therefore I will wait for Him.'" Good stuff! (If I had had italics capability, I would have italicized part of that. You can put your own in.)

Sometimes Dick has affliction, and his soul and everything else about him is pretty (very) downcast the days of his chemo treatments, but he is not consumed. He is in the middle of his two weeks off of treatments (so it is actually three weeks between treatments) before he starts on his second of four rounds, so he is actually feeling quite good right now. He is taking Paxil and has an appointment with a (Christian) psychologist for the day before his next treatment. He is also going to be driven into Boston by a very fine retired GENLTEman from church, so hopefully these things will help.

Jeremy sounds extremely busy - as in 6-8 hrs a day in the studio for architecture projects. One project was bashed by his professor after 20 hrs work, but after a total of 80 hrs (I'm not sure; this might have been a joint project) it was praised. He says he has time for NOTHING except architecture. He does have a job washing dinner dishes in the fraternity, 'cause supplies are so expensive for this design course.

Zach spends most of his time doing soccer and homework. He made the varsity team, but ended up playing a total of only 10 minutes in the first 4 games (combined). Thankfully the coach put him down to JV, so now he plays most of the game. He's glad, and so am I! Still doesn't know what he wants to study in college, but his favorite course this year is Lego Logo - actually a programming course.

I'm fine - just busy.

    Love,
    Nance

****

November 11, 1999

This second round of chemo is turning out to be rougher than the chemotherapy following Dick's first cancer surgery. After the first treatment, when I went in with him, he went by himself a few times. The nausea was bad, and he became very depressed the night before each time he was to go for the next treatment. I remembered Dr. Bleday saying to us, when he told us that Dick would need another course of chemotherapy, that "even the most resilient people" can be troubled by this kind of a diagnosis, and that Dick might want to consider taking

108

some medication for depression. Dick had spoken to Dr. Huberman, the oncologist, about this and had started taking Paxil, but at this point he was so "down" that I felt something different had to happen before the next chemo treatment. He had gotten to the point where he felt nauseous just walking into the building where the chemotherapy was given.

So, without any objection from Dick, I made two phone calls. First, I called the psychologist he had seen in the past when dealing with work frustration. He agreed that it would be good for Dick to talk with someone, especially since he was already on medication for depression. He made an appointment for the day before the next treatment and another one for a few weeks later.

The second call I made was to Al, a retired gentleman from our church, to see if he might be willing to drive Dick in for his next chemotherapy appointment. Al readily agreed, and has continued to drive him for each appointment since then. It wasn't until after he had begun the driving that I realized what I had asked of him: he is 75 years old, and he lives south of us, making the trip into Boston more than an hour each way for him. I think that God did not allow me to think it through before I asked him, or I might not have done it. Nonetheless, Dick and I both feel that having Al drive has made a huge difference. The combination of having company for the long trips and taking Paxil has made Dick much less depressed.

The nausea has also improved. At first Dr. Huberman prescribed some "big guns" medicine - Kytril - which cost $42 a pill! Dick promptly vomited the first one he took, and another one later on. Since then, he has been taking Decadron (a steroid) and Ativan as well as Kytril after every treatment and he has been doing much better. He is still tired for a day or two after each treatment, but has been bouncing back a little more quickly. He has also started to gain some weight.

One negative thing has been that this ileostomy has not been as good as the last one. My guess (and it is only a guess) is that since it was expected to be quite temporary, the surgical resident did it instead of Dr. Bleday, so it just doesn't have the fine workmanship of the first one; it sticks out farther, and perhaps because of that, "accidents" (the bag coming off) have been much more common than with the first ileostomy. However, as before, Dick's attitude is exemplary; he just deals with it.

****

December, 1999
    We received this manuscript from Ray.
                WE HAVE A GOOD FAMILY
    *My Mom said - when she was 83, living in an assisted living
apartment, sometimes having trouble finding the right words - "We have
a good family." As she lost words and lost the ability to remember, she
didn't lose her mind. The constraints of lost words forced on her an
elegant simplicity. As she was losing what she needed to take care of
herself, and Dad (to compensate?) was stiffening in his habits, neither
lost their personality. Mom was right: we have a good family.*
    *I always knew that it was good, if good meant "not bad". We had no
divorces in the immediate family, no black sheep, no drug abusers or
perverts, no "failures". We were all educated, respectable, and stable;
we were all Christians. But in mid-life my sisters showed me a deeper
level of that goodness.*
Part I
    *It started when Dick, my younger sister's husband, got cancer. The
facts, at the beginning, were simple. Dick, at age 47, had an episode of
rectal bleeding. A scope revealed a small cancer low in the rectum.
When the Harvard-based colorectal surgeon did a resection and
anastamosis, two of the five lymph nodes removed were positive for
cancer - showing the cancer had begun to spread. Dick was scheduled
for radiation and chemotherapy, and told he had a 60% chance of cure.
It is undoubtedly troubling to have cancer, especially when the odds of
being alive in five years are not much greater than getting heads when
flipping a coin. That alone would be enough background for the rest of
my story. But the facts, and the course of Dick's disease, did not remain
simple.*
    *Dick developed severe diarrhea post-operatively, a complication of
the antibiotics given during surgery. Then he had an abscess behind the
rectum which needed draining. Fever and pain continued, and further
studies revealed a leak in the anastamosis. He had an ileostomy,
improved, and took chemotherapy. After it was finished, he had his
intestines hitched up again. A routine colonoscopy done a year after the
first showed another new cancer, higher up in the colon. He had surgery
again, and again two out of five lymph nodes were positive. He was re-
hospitalized once for post-operative pain, and eventually begun on a new
schedule of chemotherapy. No one attempted to specify his odds of cure
with a percent figure; no one knew.*

Since this is not a story about medical science, it is not important to dissect these facts and analyze the course of his cancers. The simple version, "Dick has cancer", is enough for the beginning of my story. I assumed that when my sister Nancy met me at Boston's airport for my first visit after hearing about the cancer, we would both look at each other through mutual films of tears, and then she'd collapse in my arms. We don't do that sort of thing very often in our family, but it had happened, and I sort of figured it would again. It didn't. Her concerns were the usual: good to see us, a few cute jokes, was our trip OK?, and how was she going to get out of the airport parking garage. We talked about Dick some in the car - he's had a rough time, but things are getting better. Can I change lanes now? No, we don't know it will all turn out, so we're taking life one day at a time. No melodrama, just the facts. The same with Dick when we got home: Welcome. Good to see you. I'm doing OK; feeling a lot better this week. The facts.

But during that first visit, I saw something beyond the facts, something I wasn't expecting. We always laugh there, but it seemed that this week our laughter was fuller. Dick made more jokes. Nancy was never morose. After his first chemotherapy treatment, Dick drove with us to an Ethiopian restaurant where we ate with both his sons and their girlfriends. Then we got a movie to watch. Dick was part of everything. I think the "something beyond" I was seeing was joy. Joy that he may be dead in five years? No, precisely the converse: joy that he wasn't dead now, a joy Nancy shared fully. This was no "brave front", no defense mechanism, not a denial that death may be far closer than any of us could bear to think about.

The next summer, after the second cancer, the joy was still there. One evening, just as dinner was ending, he made a rather wild witty remark as he was leaving the table. I commented on it to his son Zach who said, "Yeah, Dad's getting kind of raucous." I'd noticed, I said. How come? "Oh, it's ever since the cancer." Dick himself told me that if he was only going to be alive for five more years, he thought he might start riding a motorcycle again. A death wish? No, he loved life too much for that, and his family, and his job. He simply wanted to live life fully, and riding a motorcycle - carefully, without crashing it - was one way to do that.

Nancy had told me several times that they could only live life one day at a time. How odd: it takes having cancer to discover, or at least to articulate, the obvious. And it took their cancer to show me joy.

Part II
(Editorial note: part II is not our story, and as Aslan says in the Narnia Series by C. S. Lewis, you shouldn't tell some else's story).
Conclusion
We have a good family; my sisters showed me how good.

****

December, 1999
Christmas letter
This year in my letter I recounted the story about the man who was stranded on the island and how the smoke from his burned hut attracted a passing ship. I used the story as a framework for telling about the events in the Klines' lives over the past twelve months. I ended the letter as follows:
In some sense, the ship hasn't arrived for us yet. Dick still has 3 months of chemo left, and then he faces another surgery for closure of the ileostomy - probably around March. However, we're really enjoying the island, and more and more we are confident that something which seems so devastating can be used in God's hands to be better than anything we could imagine.
The bottom line is, that Baby, who was born 2000 years ago, was and is the Answer to every problem we have ever had or will have. Let's rejoice in His coming and remember as we start the new year Whose birth started the calendar in the first place!
Merry Christmas to you.

Thunder:

January 2000

Chapter 15

January 15, 2000
Email from Dick to about 15 of our friends
Title: "And the Ship Hit an Iceberg",

So the captain picked me up after he saw my smoke signals (from my hut burning down) and we sailed out into the beautiful South Pacific seas. We traveled for several hundred miles for several days and it was beautiful, especially after being isolated for so long. But then, in the middle of the night, the ship suddenly hit a rogue iceberg that had drifted down from the North Atlantic seas. The iceberg ripped open the side of the ship below the water line, and the ship started to list greatly to one side. To my uninformed mind, I started to think, "This is it, the ship is going down; we're all shark bait now." But once again, I doubted the Captain. He knew how to handle the ship. The ship is still listing to one side, but we have stopped taking on water and the ship is steaming slowing back to the island, a safe place. The difference is that this time we have a radio and the Captain has already sent out a call for another ship to come pick us up. The Captain is not worried.

Many of you received our Christmas letter this year, and for those who had the time to read it, you will recognize the above as a continuation of that letter. For those who didn't receive it, or else didn't have time to read it, the above probably doesn't make much sense, for which I apologize. I'll fill you in on the real details below. I want to thank everyone on this email list for your many prayers during the past two years. Things have changed in the past few days, and this email is an SOS requesting your continued prayers. Some of you already know some of the details and have already been praying, and as the above indicates, things are looking somewhat better than at first. (Your prayers are already being answered).

It all started around Thanksgiving time. This was a good time in that it was an off time from the chemotherapy, so I was feeling good during the holiday and enjoyed the time with family and friends. One problem that I had a few times during those latter weeks, though, was some headaches and blurred vision. I didn't tell anyone about it at the time (even Nancy), but when I returned to start the next round of chemo in December, I told my oncologist about the problems. He said that since it was during the off time, that it was probably not related to the chemo, but rather was episodes of migraine headaches.

During the month of December, during the next round of chemo, I didn't have any more problems with vision or headaches, so both my oncologist and I were relatively at ease with his initial diagnosis of the problem. Then Christmas and the new year arrived. Once again, it was a joyous time. I was off the chemo again for several weeks - not that they take you off chemo for the holidays, but my cycles just happened to fall with the off times during the holidays. Jeremy has been "home" from Virginia these weeks, as has Liz (our niece from Kenya who is going to BU and stays with us during the holidays). Their presence and visiting friends and family have all resulted in a great fun, blessed time. But again during the off time from the chemo I had worse headaches and worse episodes of blurred vision.

I returned to start the fourth and last round of chemo a week ago Friday (yesterday). As it turns out, I didn't have chemo that day because my blood counts were too low from the previous round of chemo. My oncologist decided that we would wait another week and start the chemo at that time (i.e., yesterday) if I was ready. However, I told him again of the continuing, and worsening episodes during the off times. He decided that we should be proactive and said he would schedule me for an MRI (a brain scan) as soon as possible.

On Wednesday morning I received a phone call at work that there was a slot available on the machine in the afternoon. I drove into Boston and had the brain scan. I still wasn't too worried about the outcome. It really helps to know where you're going (i.e., home in heaven) even though you don't know the details (i.e., when or how).

The phone call from my oncologist came later Thursday afternoon at work. The MRI showed a tumor in the brain (an assumed metastasis from the colon cancer). He felt it was important that we stop the chemo immediately and treat the brain tumor aggressively now! He had already set up an appointment for me on Friday morning at 8:30 with a neurosurgeon at the Deaconess. He strongly suggested that "your wife would want to be there as well".

Needless to say, Nancy took yesterday off from work, and we spent much of yesterday at the hospital: seeing the neurosurgeon first thing; seeing my oncologist to update him and have further discussions on the steps from here; my primary health care physician (PCP) to obtain the necessary referrals for the neurosurgeon, MRI's, etc., and to have a repeat MRI in the afternoon to get a closer, more detailed look at the *tumor and to do a more comprehensive search for other possible lesions in the brain.*

Backing up a little, things appeared pretty bleak to us Thursday evening. I was ready to throw in the towel, depending upon what the neurosurgeon said the next morning. The bleakest time for me was the first few moments in the office. He pulled no punches: I have a two centimeter (slightly under one inch, for you non metric types) tumor deep in the cerebellum. He threw the MRI images up on the light box. There it was, no mistaking, even my untrained eyes could clearly see it. It looked very large to my eyes, and very deep in the brain. I silently said to myself, "Well this is it. I'm going home".

However, from that point on, as we discussed the possibilities for treatment, things started to look up. It turns out that if you have a brain tumor, the cerebellum is a good place to have it. Even though it is "in there", they can create an incision in the brain and get at it to surgically remove it all, and although there are possible complications, as with any surgery, the risk is considered small, almost routine. I should recover rapidly from the surgery. It's expected that I will only need to spend about two nights in the hospital and then after about one month recovery period, start radiation. I will have six weeks of full brain radiation afterwards, which will probably be worse than the actual brain surgery. I may lose some coordination in my left hand after surgery, but this should be temporary (four to six weeks). Worst case is that I might develop a tremor in my left hand/arm after surgery, and if so, this will probably be permanent; but again, this is not expected, only possible.

There were two possible treatments for the tumor, but since this letter is already much too detailed and long, I will spare you those details. But one thing I do want to say is that the neurologist we were talking to Friday morning explained everything to us and said "I can do this, and everything will probably come out all right". However, in talking about the different possibilities for treatment, at the end he said he would like to get the opinion of the chief of neurosurgery, who happened to be in surgery at the time. So the three of us walked from his office over to the hospital. Nancy and I waited outside in the waiting room while the doctor suited up and walked into the operating room with my scans to discuss it with the chief of neurosurgery. When he came out of the operating room, he said that the chief neurologist agreed with our joint decision that surgery was the best option, and not only that, but the chief neurologist will do the surgery. I have an appointment to see the chief neurologist this coming Tuesday afternoon.

Lastly, the repeat MRI Friday afternoon showed two things. One, it is not a single tumor, but two separate tumors that are very close together. The neurologist explained on the phone (Friday evening) that they would still probably be able to remove both tumors at the same time, but maybe not. We will find out more Tuesday. The second is that no other lesions appeared in the scan. This is good! The whole brain radiation afterwards is to hopefully kill any lesions which are too small to show up.

Also, the reason that the headaches and blurred vision didn't show up during the chemo was that during the chemo cycles I was on a steroid (for nausea), and the steroid decreases the swelling in the brain and therefore masks the problem. The good thing about this is that I'm now on the same steroid for the brain tumor and haven't been having problems (today!). Too bad this couldn't be a permanent solution, but I'll take what I can get.

Jeremy heads back to Virginia tomorrow (Sunday). Pray for him. This is difficult for him, leaving me and the family, just when we are about to enter into another period of trials. Pray that he will have peace, concentrate on his studies, and know that it is all right to be absent physically. We know that he is with us in prayer and concern. Pray also for Nancy and Zachary; these times are whole family affairs.

Well, that's just about everything we know at this point. Again, thanks for your many prayers, and please don't stop. And for those of you that had the patience to read through this entire email, job well done and thanks again.

> *God bless you all,*
> *Dick*

****

January 17, 2000

If we had any doubts that our friends were interested in our lives, they are gone now. We keep receiving very loving and encouraging cards and notes and we are now receiving a flood of emails in response to the one Dick sent a couple of days ago. These are parts of some of them to Dick or me or both of us.

From Anne (an old friend and the wife of Dick's best man):
I thank God that you are in my life - and indeed that we are part of each other FOREVER. I'll step up the prayers again, from once a week

117

(Tuesdays!) to "on the alert" (i.e. waking up in the night, "feeling" a nudge, etc.) Call anytime day or NIGHT if we can pray or help. Truly. Nothing worse than middle of the night fears when you're the only one awake!

I send much, much love, with the peace that the One who holds you in His arms loves you (and yours) even more than WE do!!!

From Marcia (a good friend and coworker of mine):

I didn't know if you would feel like talking on the phone so I just wanted to send this to let you know that I'm thinking of you. If you feel like talking give me a call. (I think this might be the third e-mail I've ever sent - I hope it works!)

From Tim (the director of the camp where Zach worked):

I ask God for many things for you. One is that ten or twenty years from now, you and Nancy will look back on these days and think "Those were tough times - glad they're over."

Keep trusting God even when you don't understand Him. Lots of us are praying for you.

From Scott (a friend with whom we both lived in Christian community in 1974-1975):

Thank you for the update. This is a hard thing. Life seems to require more courage than I ever imagined it would, sometimes just to keep going. There have been times when I didn't think I could keep going, and I longed for a legitimate way out. It appears to me that you have had enough courage to keep on, to keep fighting, not just for yourself, but for the people who care about you, which includes me among all the others. That was important to me - at times when I wanted to die, I realized that even if I didn't want to live for me, there were a number of other people who cared about me, and who would have been devastated had I chosen not to go on living. And because I loved those people, I would go on.

I have been reflecting the past couple of days on something I heard a while ago, somewhere, perhaps it was Solzhenitsyn. In effect, it went "God's purpose is not that we should live nice lives, his purpose is the formation of our souls". . . There is a perspective there that goes beyond this world.

From Ray:

When Mike and Lisa got married in Knoxville a few months before we did, the pastor said, "You are not getting married for yourselves. You are getting married for others." It was a sentiment I hadn't heard before, but somehow felt it fit for Jan and me - and maybe for all marriages. Well, (and you probably already know this) this cancer business is not just for you (to bear, to learn from, to wrestle with). It is for all of us. We are carrying it with you. But even more, we are blessed (an old word deserving resurrection now and then) in watching and being part of your faith; we are in awe of God's work in you.

From Bob (the dear friend who married us):

Dick, I appreciate your honesty and candor in the email. You spoke openly and candidly about your fears going through this diagnostic process. I respect you tremendously for your candor. I trust you will be able to continue the honesty as you go through the next stretch of treatment. . .

May I end with my favorite benediction from The Book of Common Prayer (being a good Episcopalian).

The peace of God, which passeth all understanding, keep your hearts and your minds in the knowledge and love of God, and of His Jesus Christ our Lord; and the blessing of God Almighty, the Father, the Son, and the Holy Ghost, be amongst you and remain with you always. Amen.

I've spent a lot of time pondering that benediction, and I think it has a lot to say to us. I hope you find it as meaningful as I do.

From Beth (my college roommate):

Thank you for caring enough about us to share with us your darkest news, and your brightest hopes. I have thought about you almost constantly since reading your email Sunday morning. . .

Dick, you have Nancy and your wonderful sons at your side, and you have a great Captain guiding your ship. For this I am very thankful. As a friend from afar, I tell you that I will support you all in any way that I can. And, you are in my prayers throughout the day. I sense a chorus of voices rising to heaven asking for restoration of health for your earthly body. I can almost hear the cacophony of sound. I've never sensed that before.

The kind of support we have been receiving from both near and far is certainly a tremendous gift at this time. It definitely makes us feel less alone.

****

January 19, 2000
Email from Dick to about 30 friends and relatives
Title: "The Heavens are telling of the Glory of God (or don't forget your pants)"
An update:
First, thank you. We have been overwhelmed with the outpouring of love and support since sending out our first email. The emails have been returning daily and opening each one has been like opening up a special package at Christmas, reading the kind words of love and support. I wish we had had the time to answer each one, but as you might guess, a lot has been going on.
I hope you noticed my subject line above. I'll repeat it just in case you missed it: "The Heavens are telling of the Glory of God (or don't forget your pants)."
It seems like I always have to make things difficult; can't just be normal like everyone else. I'm afraid we have had some more difficult times since our previous email. As related previously, things were beginning to look up a little bit. The last information was that there were the two tumors in the cerebellum which were close together and it was hopeful that both could be removed surgically with hopefully little risk. That was Friday.
On Sunday evening (the coldest night in Massachusetts in three years!) I started to get a stiff neck, so I decided to go to bed early. My neck became increasingly worse during the night until I couldn't stand the pain any longer and woke Nancy up around 4:00 a.m. She called the neurosurgeon at the hospital (resident) and he indicated that we should come into the hospital right away. Nancy woke Zach up to help drive me in, but it became clear to me that I couldn't move (i.e., couldn't get out of bed because of the pain in my neck when I tried to move my head at all). I told Nancy that she needed to call an ambulance.
The Walpole rescue squad came and did their thing to slide me on to a portable, backboard stretcher and with great difficulty down the stairs and out into the cold night air to the ambulance. I remember thinking "Why is this happening to me?", but at the same time I

remember that on that very cold night while being carried across the front yard that the sky was crystal clear and that the heavens were absolutely beautiful, and it helped to remind me about God's great love for His children.

The local rescue squad transported me to Norwood hospital where I was stabilized with Decadron (a steroid for swelling), a neck brace, and morphine, and then another ambulance transported me to Beth Israel Hospital where they did further tests (MRI and X-ray) of the neck looking for the cause. Unfortunately, they have found another abnormality (I'm growing to hate that phrase) in my neck. Although the resident on Monday morning said it _might_ be another tumor, the neurosurgeon that we saw Tuesday said it probably _is_ another (third) tumor.

So the three of us (Zach, Nancy, and myself) spent the wee hours of Monday morning and most of Monday in the emergency room at Beth Israel Hospital. Luckily for me, Nancy and Zach are not without a good sense of humor, and despite the problems and uncertainty, there were many almost fun moments together as a family.

One such moment was when we realized that they were thinking of releasing me, since my condition had improved considerably, and that I didn't have any shoes, socks, or pants. Indeed, when the rescue squad carried me out the front door of our house, I was wearing exactly what I was sleeping in: undershorts, a tee shirt that said "Walpole Post Prom Party, Up All Night at the YMCA", and that was it. We had unpleasant mental pictures of me walking out through the lobby of the hospital into the cold air in my scant wardrobe. They did release me Monday afternoon. Luckily, the COOP was open just a block down from the hospital and Nancy, being a good egg, ran down and bought me a pair of pants, and being so cold, Zach had two jackets and was kind enough to lend me one. And the hospital gave me a pair of socks so at least I didn't have to walk out into the cold with bare feet! And thus, "don't leave home without your pants!"

On Tuesday we had our meeting with the chief neurosurgeon at Beth Israel Deaconess Hospital. It is not clear whether he will be able to remove the small tumor in the cerebellum because it is small and very deep in, so finding it is the problem. He will go for it first. If he can't find it, then they will treat later on with radiation. He will then remove the second tumor in the cerebellum which is both larger and closer to the surface, so therefore much easier to find. The possible tumor in the neck, it that's what it is, will have to be dealt with at a later time, through conventional radiation therapy.

121

Schedule and prayer requests:
1) I am scheduled for a whole body bone scan tomorrow (Thursday). Three tumors is enough as far as I'm concerned, so please pray that no more tumors show up on the scan.
2) I have a pre-op physical Monday (standard fare before surgery).
3) Surgery is scheduled for Wednesday, starting at 9:30 a.m. Pray that the surgeon would be able to remove both brain tumors and that there would not be subsequent complications requiring extended hospitalization and/or extensive rehabilitation.
A final word of insight that we have gained through this. A rare gem expressed by our friend Tom in one of our Tuesday night home Bible studies: "We shouldn't put our faith in the answer to our prayers, but rather in the One who causes the outcome."
God bless,
Dick
P.S. thanks for letting me ramble on.

****

January 20, 2000
We continue to receive so many wonderful emails and cards.
This is part of an email from Don (a friend formerly of Walpole, now living in Connecticut)
My sympathies of the new news and another ordeal to wade through. How great it is that you can do so with love, hope and laughter. You can truly feel the spirit of Christ in your story.
It has been and must be a difficult time for you. However, when I am drifting off at night - dreaming yet or not, I don't know - and my thoughts turn to you, it is often of a party. Yes, a wild party in which we are praising God - shouting and singing to His glory! The reason for all this is not because you have "gone" HOME, but because He has allowed you to stay in your temporary home. I am (we are) definitely walking, straining, hoping and praying with you in this valley, but for some reason I can't get this picture of the celebration that comes after out of my head. We look forward to participating in the celebration of His grace and mercy with you one day soon - which is not to minimize your current struggles, but I guess their magnitude only gives reason to the intensity of the future celebration.
May God keep you all, and continue to fill with His love, peace, patience and joy.

This came from Ray. He sent the words to a song by Michael Kelly Blanchard, and I was particularly struck by the last two stanzas:

God, your mercy found us.
Faithfulness surrounds us
Priceless grace has bound us
To the cross of...

Thy true love,
Standing in a world of toppled dreams,
Shining in the swirl of in-betweens,
The light still beams
From thy true love.

From Beth:

Your situation is a wake-up call for me, to remember the gift of life. May every day be precious in our sight. I can't make it better, no matter how hard I try. I think I have spent most of my motherhood thinking I could somehow control outcomes and make them better on my own. I can't, but you have reminded me Who can.

Chapter 16

January 21, 2000
Email from Dick to friends
Title: "Prayer #1 --> Answered!!! :-)"
The Bone scan did not show any more tumors. One anomaly on my chin, but this could be from former dental work. Something to "look at" later, but nothing else showed up in the rest of my bones that was of concern to the radiology resident that was there to interpret the results. Therefore, since the scan was clear (i.e., they would not have put me through brain surgery if other tumors were prevalent in my bones), surgery is on for Wednesday morning, 9:30.
Thanks for your prayers,
Dick

****

January 23, 2000
A package arrived for me today. It was one of those Next Day Delivery things, so I had to sign for it. It was from Anne, and it had cost her over $18 to mail it, so I knew it was important, but I couldn't figure what it could be until I read the note she had enclosed: "Friday AM. What oh what can I DO that will let Nancy know how <u>much</u> I love her and am thinking of her. . . ? The answer that came to me is enclosed. <u>XOXOX</u>. Anne" The note gave it away. I just knew it was fudge. Anne makes the best fudge in the world, and though she had tried once to teach me, I never have been able to make it as good as she does. This batch is no exception: about a pound of fudge, just poured out and not even cut. Since it was addressed specifically to me, I don't think she intends for me to share it very much. . .

****

January 25, 2000
Email from Dick to Anne
Thanks for your emails, prayers, and support during this time. The chocolate fudge was delicious, what little I had. Nancy would beat us off

with a baseball bat whenever Zach or I would approach. It was absolutely vicious at times.

****

January 25, 2000
Email from Dick to friends
Title: "On Schedule with God's Divine Providence"
A quick note, and then some more therapeutic rambling.

Things are going according to schedule, so therefore Nancy and I will be hopefully arriving at the hospital tomorrow morning (Wednesday) at 8:00 for my 9:30 operation. I realize the operation will be over before most of you read this email, but I also know that you will be praying for us. Thanks!

We were originally wondering about this snow storm, whether it would cause some sort of delay, but in God's divine providence the storm has moved through the region quicker than originally expected and it appears that we should hopefully not have any serious problems traveling in the morning.

Thanks to all again for your many caring emails and phone calls and your many words of encouragement. Nancy and I want you all to know the extreme peace that we both feel. It truly is a peace that passes all understanding, something that is not from within ourselves, but something that God has given us as a special measure of faith at the present. This past weekend, especially, we really enjoyed together as a family and were truly almost giddy at times with joy and laughter.

The peace we are feeling is truly in the very nature of God. By this, I don't mean that we have God all figured out and that we understand what's going on here. We don't know what the outcome will be, but we are confident that we are experiencing God's divine providence: that He knows what's going on here, and that whatever happens it is best for me (Dick), Nancy, our family, and our friends (you!).

A couple of scripture passages that I have been recently reflecting upon:

James 1:13b, 17 - "...for God cannot be tempted by evil, and He Himself does not tempt any one... Every good thing bestowed and every perfect gift is from above, coming down from the Father of lights, with whom there is no variation, or shifting shadow."

I might be taking the first part slightly out of context, but what it says to me is that no evil thing ever comes from God; it's just not possible; it's not consistent with His perfect nature ("with whom there is no variation, or shifting shadow!"), but rather every good thing comes from God. We need to understand this even when things seem rough and difficult at times, that God has the big picture in mind and that He can only do what is the loving and perfect thing - the divine providence of God. I'm not saying it very well (remember, I'm an engineer, not a poet or theologian), but it is a fact that God has impressed on our hearts, and Nancy and I wanted you all to know of His grace in our lives at this time so you wouldn't be worrying about us.

Isaiah 55:9 - "As the heavens are higher than the earth, so are my ways higher than your ways and my thoughts higher than your thoughts." - God's divine providence.

And one of Nancy's favorite verses these past several weeks:

Phil 4:4,7 - "Rejoice in the Lord always. I will say it again: Rejoice! . . . Do not be anxious about anything, but in everything, by prayer and petition, with thanksgiving, present your requests to God. And the peace of God, which transcends all understanding, will guard your hearts and your minds in Christ Jesus." Thanks for standing by us,

> *Love to you all,*
> *Dick and Nancy*

****

January 26, 2000

The alarm went off at 5:30 this morning, and I thought it was yet another fire alarm at my school; that would make it the fourth in four days. Then I realized with some relief that it was not a fire alarm but the alarm waking me up to get ready to go in for Dick's brain surgery.

For some reason, despite the peace I have been experiencing - I guess in the middle of the peace - I've had numerous thoughts that Dick could die during this surgery. It's quite unreasonable - more likely that he will go through the surgery fine and have more treatments after - with some completely unknown outcome. Nonetheless, I just felt compelled to ask him last night - for future reference - about his funeral wishes. He would like Bob Ludwig and Paul Scaringi to lead a memorial service. Great idea. I hadn't thought of them. Maybe if I go first, they could do my service, too. He says he wants to give his body to science (Harvard Medical School) but first have it for calling hours and a memorial service. I said that seemed dumb - having to buy a casket for just a couple of days, since we wouldn't be putting it in the ground, but he says we could borrow a casket. (<u>Borrow</u> a casket?!?)

Anyway, we have both felt quite peaceful; we had a quiet ride into the hospital, but not morose. All was fine until the good-bye kiss when he went to the prep room. As he walked away, I could see he was starting to cry. Darn! I'm glad I am alone in this waiting room - listening to Caedmon's Call on my new Discman. Caedmon's Call is a fairly new group with a really nice sound and more thought provoking words than most. Thought provoking can be tear-producing, too, but that's okay. I haven't had a good cry in a while. Now is as good a time as any, I guess. I'll probably have a long wait. Funny; I just heard the singer sing "cold in Kansas City" and it sounded to me like "colon cancer". Life looks so different now - even <u>sounds</u> different.

****

January 26, 2000 - end of the day
Email to friends:
DEAR Friends,

Just a quick update from the other half. I don't feel particularly creative or eloquent at the moment, but I wanted to thank you all for your many prayers and much appreciated notes. What an OVERWHELMING outpouring of support! The surgery was long but successful. The surgeon (who the admitting nurse said this am is "one of the best neurosurgeons in the country") said that he was able to remove both tumors, and with not too much cutting of brain tissue, so that rehabilitation shouldn't be a problem. When I left Dick this evening, he was clear mentally and his repeated neurological checks were fine. All limbs were working well (in bed, of course). He had a bad headache, though he was sleeping most of the time in between feeling the headache. The good news from the resident is that these headaches are normal. The bad news is that they can last for a week or two!

The other good news is that I called the hospital when I got home and the ICU nurse said that Dick said the med she had given him helped and he was feeling much better. Praise God! He will be in ICU - as a matter of course - until probably mid day tomorrow, then to a regular floor, if all goes well.

For those of you who have been concerned about me, your prayers are much appreciated. I packed my backpack last night planning to hunker down with books and CD's for the long haul. I started in the

127

waiting room by myself - started with a good cry and got that over with and got on with writing in my journal etc. To my great surprise and delight, mid-morning brought three dear and generous friends to sit with me through the day. The time passed far more quickly and pleasantly than it would have had I been by myself.

I don't look forward to driving in and out of Boston to the hospital, but, as Dick says, "You just have to DRIVE, and when you get there, you get there!" That's sort of how I'm looking at this whole big experience. Yesterday my school celebrated School Nurse Day for me (talk about good timing!) and one of my gifts was a gift certificate for a complete house cleaning. How's that for being cared for?

Okay, so I never could get by with just a few words. I'll try better next time. Continued prayers would not be refused.

Okay. One more thing. This is how I see prayer (for those of you who haven't already heard this). It's like Burger King vs. a gourmet restaurant. We go to Burger King to "have it your way" - a burger, no onions, large shake, medium fries, successful surgery, no complications, complete healing , please. We know just what we want. But prayer is like going to a gourmet restaurant. We see that the prices are quite steep, so we just order an appetizer - mozzarella sticks. But then the maitre d' comes and says that we will be getting the chef's special. We may or may not get the mozzarella sticks, but the point is, we get the chef's BEST. In the prayer sense, the BEST is "peace that transcends all understanding". Maybe we'll get the other stuff we're seeking - maybe not, but we get the BEST.

> *Love,*
> *Nancy*

****

January 27, 2000
Email from me to friends
Title: "Good Progress"
Hello everybody!

Truly QUICK note this time.

Dick is doing well! Headaches seem much improved. He had gone five and a half hours without pain med when I left him this evening. He walked the halls with me twice(!) He ate all his meals today - glad that they did not put him on a bland diet like they did for the other surgeries.

I was a little down and tired this am, but reading the emails that some of you sent really perked me up. (And don't feel bad if you didn't send one; I wouldn't have had time to read any more before work.)

Both Jeremy and Zach talked to Dick in the hospital and felt obviously good about that.

Love to you all - Good night!

Nancy

****

January 28, 2000

Another gem among our treasure of emails, from Carole (a friend from our days in Christian community in the 1970's):

I keep thinking of the scripture in 1John: "God is light and in God there is no darkness at all. If we (choose to) walk in the light we have fellowship with one another (and ourselves and God) and the blood of Jesus purifies us from all sin."

I think about how you and Dick have chosen to see God in every step of this journey; you have chosen to look for the light, to shine the light in the darkness, to step into the light, to let the light heal and transform, and in so doing, you have led us into the light with you. Thank you for sharing this journey with us, and being a teacher to all of us as you have been so faithful to God and one another.

****

January 29, 2000

Zach and I went in to see Dick yesterday, arriving around 4:45 PM. Two friends were visiting him when we arrived, and after they left, Dick seemed a little down, with sort of a flat affect. He said he felt sort of weird - like he would do something, but then not feel as though he had done it - like he had to "press the reset button." He said it was like an "out of body" experience. He also seemed rather humorless (which is particularly difficult for me). He was a little sharp with both Zach and me on a couple of occasions, and less affectionate than usual. All in all, it wasn't my best visit with him. I got home and found I had nothing to say in an email, so I decided not to write one. This morning, in pursuit of honesty, I considered writing one and simply saying that Dick was "a little down", but I was effectively blocked from doing that because with six different attempts to reach my email server, I could not get on the internet.

Bobbie called this morning to ask how things were going. I ended up venting my concerns to her. She felt that a lot of Dick's flat affect could be from the muscle relaxant that he has been taking, and the "out of body" experience was a complaint that she had had from some of her patients who were on the steroid that has been prescribed for him.

So, I left to pick him up late this morning with hopes that much of his mood change was due to medications. In fact, he was much brighter, and it is such a joy to have him around again!

A few words about Zach:

1 - He's more gullible than I thought. One day we were walking through the long, stark, joyless tunnel that joins the parking garage to the hospital, and I pointed to some ominous looking chrome containers - each about five feet by three feet by three and a half feet - and I told Zach they were for dead bodies. "They are?" He was fooled only for a minute - until he saw the trays of food in an open one of the containers and also concluded that containers of this size might easily fit a body the size of his mother's, but not one any bigger!

2 - He's creative. He had me shave his head last night to 1/8 inch, leaving just a T on the top for the Tennessee Titans for the Super Bowl. We called Liz to see how we could dye the T, but having no advice from her, we used food coloring. Shortly after we did it, she called back to say, "Don't use food coloring; it doesn't come out!" (It did.)

3 - He's a good wrestler. There recently was a newspaper article highlighting one of his matches: "Marauders' Hopes de-Kline". He is nearly through the season, and for the second year in a row has not gotten pinned in a wrestling match. That is quite an accomplishment and an indicator of his strength and perseverance.

****

January 29, 2000
Email from Dick to friends
Title: "Home"
Greetings to all,

Just a note to let you know that it is Saturday afternoon and that I am home, doing well, as Nancy previously reported.

I will return Monday afternoon to have the staples removed (ouch!) and then the next big date is Monday February 7, when I will be going to

the "brain clinic" at Beth Israel Hospital where I will meet with a number of specialists to determine the course of treatment from this point.
Thanks to all,
Dick

****

January 31, 2000
Email from Jan to us
Dear Nancy and Dick,
Home after only five days? Sounds impressive to me. Thanks for keeping us up to date with all that is going on. It is also impressive to see the number of people who receive your mailings. You have people all over the world who are part of your community of faith who are praying for you. We minister to you through our prayers and you nourish our faith by showing us what God is doing in your lives. A remarkable thing! I experienced something a bit like that last July as a result of this HIV thing. I became aware of God loving me through my community of faith. That awareness has stayed with me.
I remember your mom, Nancy, once saying that she had become careful about praying for patience. Whenever she prays for patience God seems to give her plenty of things to be patient about!! I remember at the beginning of this whole cancer business asking God to show me how to pray for you, Dick. So God clobbers me with a positive HIV test. During the month of July God showed me some of the best things about myself and some of the worst things as well. I still have not recovered from the experience, but then I don't want to. I want God to keep working on me. The experience certainly did give me a better idea of how to pray for you!!
By the way, I stuck myself again in surgery a couple of days ago, the first time in over a year. By our standards it was a low risk stick - solid needle, low risk patient, going through two pairs of gloves. But it was a reminder that the risk is still there as is the risk of getting smashed up on Kenya's roads or getting severe malaria. When we came to Africa God didn't make any deals with us. He didn't promise that if we served him faithfully He would make sure none of these things would ever happen to us. The only promise I can recall is the promise He gave to all His people: "Lo, I am with you always..." But then [my Kenyan friend] Savala would say - and I know you both will agree - that covers

EVERYTHING. That is enough! To be in God's presence, to know that the Palm of His hand is our home is enough.

Dick, engineer and now both poet and theologian as well, thank you for sharing with us what God is doing in your life. It has helped put a lot of things into perspective for me.

Love,
Jan

High Winds:

February 2000 - May 2000

Chapter 17

February 2, 2000
Email from Dick to friends
Title: "Resting Comfortably"
Just a quick note to let you know that everything is going very well at the moment. In the past 48 hours my headaches and extreme stiff neck situation has changed to just some residual incision pain which I'm usually not even aware of. I'm a little tired (sleeping a lot) and I still feel quite unsteady on the feet, but this doesn't stop me from getting around much in the house.

Nancy took a day off from work Monday so that we could have them remove the staples, as my discharge papers said, but when we showed up Monday afternoon they said that "We can't remove them yet, you were operated on Wednesday." Right! Well, we will return this Friday to remove the staples.

Doctors appointments have been a moving target also. As it stands now, the next big date is Monday, February 14 when I will attend the brain tumor clinic at BI to determine the best course for adjunct therapy.

Thanks,
Dick

****

February 10, 2000
As usual, we have received a wealth of email responses to Dick's last update. This came from Jim, a person with whom we had lived in community in the 70's. Jim was new to the email list and had just recently been sent all the "group emails" at one time:

The fact of your cancer and metastases hit hard, coming all at once to me as it did. However, I am honored to join the cloud of witnesses who will be cheering you on with prayer in this time of need. I was pleased to see so many familiar names on your email prayer partners list, quite a testimony to the faithfulness of God over a span of time. . .

I was driving to work this morning, lost in thought, when I looked over and saw an 18 wheeler with the single word KLINE in huge letters on its side. I got this subtle message and began to pray for all of you.

Afterwards I laughed at God's methods. For some people a 1 inch yellow memo on the refrigerator is enough; others require...

****

February 14, 2000

Today was the Brain Tumor Clinic. Now that was interesting. It was exactly what we thought it would be in that we figured it would <u>not</u> be what we thought it would be, and it wasn't! Dick and I had both privately imagined that it would be three doctors and us sitting around a table (a heavy, large mahogany table in a conference room is what I pictured) discussing the best treatment options for Dick at this point. Not quite. First of all, we had to wait more than an hour and a half before we were seen at all, and then it was by someone (maybe a nurse or nurse's assistant?) who did not know that Dick had had surgery or really anything about him. She just took his vital signs and told him his blood pressure was VERY LOUD. She then left to "grab" one of the doctors, who finally came in about 45 minutes later. (I opted to pass the time we were waiting by playing with the doctor's reflex hammer and tuning fork, but Dick discouraged this.)

The doctor who finally came in, Dr. Tishler, was a neuro-radiologist. Dr. Tishler was very personable and suggested that Dick have the fourth cervical vertebra irradiated at the time of the whole brain radiation. This would simply be a matter of "opening the window" for the radiation, which as a matter of course would extend to the second cervical vertebra anyway.

Dr. Tishler spent a little while with us discussing the what and why of further treatment. One exchange was a bit disturbing. Dr. T asked us, "Any questions?"

Dick responded, "My brain is very important to me. I have a very technical job, and I'm wondering about the effects of the radiation on my brain."

Dr. T, after a <u>long</u> pause, his face turned slightly away, replied, "Whenever there is tumor found in the brain, we assume that there could be smaller tumors that we can't see. We <u>could</u> wait until those tumors are visible and then treat them, or we can do radiation to the whole brain to eliminate them before they are seen. We feel this is the best option." He paused again. "Regarding side effects, there can be some short term memory loss."

I asked, "Temporary or permanent?"

135

"Could be either," he answered

Fortunately, we were not left alone for very long to ponder the implications of that interchange. After Dr. Tishler left, a neurologist, Dr. Wong, came in, put the MRI pictures up on the lighted board, and proceeded to suggest that there was no reason to irradiate the fourth cervical vertebra; we could just watch that. We pointed out that we had just discussed the opposite with Dr. Tishler; Dr. Wong then agreed that it would be fine to include C-4, since Dick would already be getting the radiation to C-2.

****

Email from Dick to friends
Title: "Greetings"

Well, the 14th came and went. Here's the news.

1) CAT scan last Friday was good, nothing abnormal showed up. :-)

2) It's not clear about the abnormality in my 4th vertebrae in my neck. Looks like a possible tumor in the MRI; bone scan didn't show anything in the area. They could biopsy it to determine for sure, but this would be another surgical procedure. Consensus seems to be to "open the field" of radiation a little bit when doing the brain and get the vertebrae as well.

3) I'll start whole brain radiation next Monday (21st).

4) I report tomorrow morning at 8:00 to the radiology department to get imaged and tattooed, i.e., to get ready for the radiation and to talk to the radiologist for more specifics.

Dick

****

February 18, 2000

Dick just bought a new computer - quite a fancy one, it seems to me - and it came with a scanner. That doesn't mean much to me except that he can now send pictures over the computer. Cool! This is good for him, since he has not been able to go back to work yet, but does have some mental energy to expend. This keeps him busy in a way that is interesting for him.   ·

****

February 21, 2000
Dick sent an email about the new computer to his brother John. He received this one in reply:
All this free time, you had better be careful. If the clock on your new computer is right, you sent that email at 4:27am this morning. You probably thought I would be sleeping, but I was already out plowing, so I had a reason to be up that early. Having this much time could get expensive for you; before you know it you will probably be looking at digital cameras, and then quick time video.
I imagine about this time you are in Boston for your first treatment. I'll be thinking of you and be interested in how things go. Let me know.

Dick's reply back to John:
Actually, it [being up at night] is a side affect of the steroid Decadron which I'm taking to keep the post surgery brain swelling down through the radiation period. Has two effects:
1) Ravenous appetite, which is leading to uncontrolled eating habit, and significant weight gain.
2) I wake up for 2 to 4 hours every night. Sometimes I wake up at 12:00 (midnight), other times at 4:00 a.m. This morning I was up from 4:00 to 6:00 a.m., and then went back to bed for two hours before getting up for the first radiation treatment. But I always wake up and once I wake up there is no use just laying there in bed, so I get up. Have found that it is a great time to surf the web (fast response), plus my new computer really zips along much FASTER :-) And playing on the computer for a couple of hours does make me tired again, so that eventually I feel like going back to bed. Still wish I had a cable modem like some lucky folks I know, but the new computer has a 56K modem whereas the old computer only had a 28K modem.
The first radiation treatment went fine this morning. Longer than the others, being first appointment, consent forms, etc. Future appointments will be at 9:45 a.m., for the next four weeks, 5 days per week.
Tell me more about quick time video! (just kidding)

****

February 22, 2000
We received this letter from Dick's mother. He is so encouraged by letters like these. Her letter really spoke to him as she talked about

newly gained insights into suffering. It was especially meaningful to him because it came from his Mom.

I have been questioning God about why He lets such a good man like my son go through so much suffering for so long. It seems there is no end to what you have been enduring for nearly two years and still much more ahead of you.

You are a parent so you will understand that it would be far easier for me to bear your pain if I could do so. I have been reading the book of Job and find myself wondering if you don't feel like Job sometimes. He never wavered in his faith but did despair sometimes because of his misery. This morning I read the following in the footnotes of my Bible: "Suffering can bring a dynamic quality to life. Just as drought drives the roots of a tree deeper to find water, so suffering can drive us beyond superficial acceptance of truth to dependence on God for hope and life."

I think this profound statement will help me accept what is going on in your life. Just wanted you to know.

****

February 23, 2000
Email from Dick to friends
At this point, I am still "resting" (although I have no trouble keeping busy!) at home. There are no noticeable side affects from the radiation at this point, and shouldn't be until about the third week. Still quite tired (napping once or twice per day) and the neck is still quite sore from the operation, but nothing severe, definitely getting better each day.

****

Email from Carole to Dick
I am leading a retreat this weekend on "Joyful Living" and part of one of my talks is on "finding joy in adversity". I kept thinking of the emails that both of you have written. I was deeply touched at the time, and continue to be by your faith and trust and yes, even the sense of joy you communicate while going through such grueling times. So I'm wondering if you'd mind if I shared some of your email thoughts with this group of joy-seeking women. Amazing how many lives your life is touching. . . God works in strange and marvelous ways!

You don't have to bother to respond unless you don't want me to use the emails.

Dick's response
Carole,

This is a confirmation to me of God's leading. It is fine with me and Nancy if you share any of the emails with others at your retreat. Something I have been working on during the past several weeks has been gathering together the "whole story" of the past 2 plus years and it is almost done. Sometime next week I expect to put the entire story on our web site: www.thecia.net/users/kline

The link on our home page will be: A Story of God's Grace (a battle with Cancer). It will include all the emails as well as letters received and church testimonials and other special artifacts that have been collected during this time. Our sincere hope (I think God's leading) is that this information will be shared with others who are going through difficult situations and that they may find the information helpful in their walk through life and their walk with God.

I'll send you an email when I put it on the web site. You can give out the web site address to your joy-seeking women if you think it appropriate, and tell them to be looking for "A Story of God's Grace", or not, as you think appropriate.

****

February 25, 2000
Email from me to Ray and Jan

I'm on vacation this week - just about over now. Dick's radiation has been going okay - one out of four weeks done. I went in with him three times, Zach went today, and he went once alone. I think we're going to plan to have other people go with him for most of the rest of the treatments. Some days his lower back bothers him (old compressed L-5 disc) - and it seems he shouldn't have to drive if he doesn't feel great. On the days when he does feel good, he might as well have company. Several people have offered, and I think it sometimes makes people feel good to be able to DO something to help.

I'm doing fine, emotionally, spiritually, physically - except when little things go wrong. Dick and I talked about it yesterday. We both feel that somehow it's easier to get through the big things - the cancer diagnoses and the surgeries - than the day to day pains and complications. Last Friday - as in FRIDAY - day before weekend - and a SNOWY Friday at that - afternoon, as in PM - Dick developed abdominal bloating / discomfort. It occurred to us to suspect adhesions / ileus again, this having happened twice before, so we made him NPO [nothing by mouth] *for about the next 12 hours and delayed calling anyone. (Unlike in Africa, there is some question about whom one should call in a situation like this. His colorectal surgeon is no longer at the same hospital with all the other docs who are seeing him now.) Anyway, he had told us to try NPO for 12-18 hrs - and see if the symptoms would pass, should they occur again, which, as I just told you, they were doing (occurring). I told Dick to walk around, which he did, and then we went to bed - waking up about every 1/2 - 1 hr all night. The belly stuff got better, and he started passing gas again, but then he couldn't urinate, and he developed a low grade fever, so we suspected beginning dehydration, but there was also the possibility of UTI* [urinary tract infection], *since he had expressed pain in the kidney area earlier in the day. So he took a little tea - diuretic, then switched to Ensure - still liquid, but non-diuretic, and then he peed, but his hips and knees and ankles hurt, so I figured there was just a little gremlin which would soon exit via his toes! Anyway, all that was a bit stressful. Very good ending, by the way. He improved steadily on Saturday, the snow stopped, and he was fine enough on Sunday to watch Zach wrestle. When things go low, the up is really UP!*

Zach came in second in the sectionals for his weight class (about a dozen towns in each section) and fifth in the State Divisionals (three sections in each division, three divisions in the state.) Tomorrow he goes to All States as an alternate - we don't know yet if he'll wrestle.

Don't have an answer on this one yet. Maybe as physicians you could explain it to us. We got an itemized bill for Dick's last hospitalization (the brain surgery one) because they want us to pay $100 a day extra for a private room and insurance doesn't cover that. I called because we didn't ask for the private room, so shouldn't have to pay for it. While I was waiting to speak to someone ("All our associates are busy at this time. Please hold the line for the next available associate.") I scanned the itemized bill, which included lab tests done during surgery (e.g. sodium, whole blood - $12; glucose, whole blood - $11; semen analysis - $201) Wait, now. SEMEN ANALYSIS - $201!?! Can you give me the WHY and HOW of that one? The surgeon is away this week, but I think we'll give a call about that on Monday . . .

****

February 28, 2000
I called the neurosurgeon, and given the difficulty we have had at times reaching doctors, I was amazed to reach him and speak with him. He sounded as surprised as I was about the semen analysis, and assured me he had not done that. He figures someone punched in a wrong code. I wonder how many things like that end up getting charged to insurance and paid for, even though they were never done!

****

February 29, 2000
Email from Dick to friends
Several different people have contacted us and said that they have shared various things we have said or written with others who are struggling with similar issues / difficulties. We felt lead to "publish" on the web the entire story of the past two years. The website: www.thecia.net/users/kline contains the link "A Story of God's Grace in the Storm". This link points to an archive of emails, letters, and transcripts of audio tapes (church testimonies) from the past two years. If after viewing it, you feel it might be useful to share with someone else, please do! If not, then just ignore. Thanks.

Chapter 18

March 2, 2000
Dick scanned an old picture into the computer and sent it to Jeremy along with the following email. The picture is of Dick in his late twenties with a full head of Afro hair, a rather scruffy mustache and goatee, a big smile on his face, and a thoughtful looking little Jeremy in a yellow baby carrier on Dick's back.

A couple of things:
1) Just in case you ever thought that your Dad wasn't always proud to have you as a son, just look at this picture. My facial expression expresses it all! "This is my Son! He's great!".
2) As you know, Mom and I scrimped and saved for most of "your" lives, one of our goals being to send you guys to college. I want to say how much I appreciate that you're not blowing it on booze, parties, women, and gut courses, but it is clear that you are working very hard and making the most of your college years (i.e., making the most of this once in a lifetime opportunity.)
However, often when we talk to you, you sound exhausted. I'd like to do two things through one gesture: 1) say thanks, 2) see that you take a break and get some rest. Therefore, what I propose is the following:
A NIGHT OUT ON DAD AND MOM
I'll reimburse you (100%) up to $100 for a special night out. After you do it, just send me an email with the bill and I'll send a check. For example, maybe you would want to take Amanda to a concert / play and dinner? Just a suggestion. It's your choice what you do.

****

March 2, 2000
When the phone rang this morning I didn't hear it because I was drying my hair, so I was a bit startled to notice the light on the answering machine blinking at 7:00. The message was from Dick's mom. His dad died early this morning. He had been in a nursing home for eight years with Alzheimer's disease. Much of that time he could not walk, talk, feed himself or recognize anyone. The question at this point is not so much "why did he die?" as "why had he lived like that for so long?" In many ways it is a blessing.

Dick, Zach and I plan to leave tomorrow night to drive out to Syracuse for the memorial service on Saturday, and we'll come back on Sunday night. Dick is feeling reasonably well, and with Zach along to help with driving, I expect that - weather permitting - the trip should be okay.

****

March 3, 2000
I am so very grateful for caring medical people. Today Dick told the radiation nurse about the nagging cough he has been having. Rather than ignoring it or opting for a "wait and see" attitude, she followed up on it with the doctors, including Dr. Coviello, Dick's primary care physician. They did a chest x-ray, which reportedly was clear, and Dr. Coviello prescribed an albuterol inhaler for him. I felt really uneasy about Dick's cough and some difficulty breathing, since we were due to leave for Syracuse. I had visions of the problem being congestive heart failure, since I had not-so-pleasant memories of that when he had the C-diff in January, 1999. I called Dr. Coviello's office and said that I really needed to speak to her, since we were leaving shortly for Dick's father's funeral. The secretary let me speak to a nurse practitioner, who reportedly left a note on Dr. C's chair so that she would call me. She did call back, and was ever so understanding of my perhaps irrational fears. She agreed that Dick certainly had to take this trip, and assured me that because the chest x-ray was clear, she really thought that Dick would be okay. However, she urged us to seek medical attention in Syracuse if needed. I appreciated that she did not just "brush me off", but took time to listen and address my concerns.

****

March 9, 2000
Email to Ray and Jan from me
Title: "Embarrassing Moment"
Now Ray, I don't know if you have your father's genes as Zach and I do, and if you can relate to the story I am about to relate; and Jan, I don't know if you have ever experienced an uncontrollable laughing fit such as I am about to describe, but if you have not, you may respond as Dick did ("You have embarrassed the whole family!") when I relate the following story.

143

It was Sunday am, the day after the funeral. We decided to go to (brother) John, Susan and Grandma's church before returning to Walpole. Grandma wanted us all to sit together, so we (with a couple of strangers) were squashed together (eight people) in a pew made for six or seven. Tight fit. All went well through the sermon and singing, and then it was communion. Now in the Presbyterian church, it is not unlike the Baptist church in that the elements are all passed around and then "partaken of" at the same time. In our church, the bread happens to be Matzo, but in this church it turned out to be a little square of something not unlike a very chewy biscuit. Now I put mine in my mouth, and was thinking, "My, this certainly is CHEWY," but I just chewed and chewed and chewed, thinking this a bit humorous, but not outrageously funny, until I heard a little snicker from Zach, who was sitting (CLOSELY, as you will recall) to my left. There was little doubt in my mind as to the reason for his snicker. (Yes, he too, had found the bread a bit chewy, and had in fact looked up to see if other parishioners were still chewing, which, in fact, they were.) Mind you, I did not look at him AT ALL. Well, as I said, on my own, this situation was a little funny, but not hilarious, but when confronted with someone who ALSO saw humor in it, one of those little bubbles of laughter floated up and came OUT MY MOUTH. Of course this was dreadful, because it was COMMUNION, for Pete's sake, and it might have even stopped then, but when Zach realized that HE was not the ONLY one who found it humorous, a big globule of laughter came out of him, and then it sort of passed back and forth. I tried ever so hard to not laugh - biting my lip and what not, but to no avail. Thinking Zach was having a coughing or crying fit, Grandma gave him a tissue, which was fortunate, because when another big clump of laughter managed to pop out when the communion grape juice was in his mouth, the tissue served to catch it.

If either of you have ever had one of these laughing fits, you may understand that the laughter is truly NOT a FUN thing at this point; one will do almost anything to stifle the laugh, which makes its untimely escape from one's person a very unpleasant sounding emission. One also works up quite a sweat with the effort to squelch the laughter, making ones wish that they were NOT the MIDDLE TWO people in the crowded pew, making any escape virtually impossible.

I think Grandma understood a bit - at least the part about the uncontrolled laughter; it happened to her a couple of times when she was pregnant. Also, I do think Richard has forgiven us. He's a good man, you know. I've already spoken to our father - to blame him for the genes that didn't include a laughter turn off button! Mary Ellen suggested it might have been an "emotional release". I'm not sure if that explains why Zach and I both feel compelled to relate this story to others, and start laughing again every time we do!

****

March 11, 2000
Ray's email response
Often when I get your messages I laugh - sometimes out loud - then I too try (as you claim to have in church) to stifle the laugh because I'm thinking, "Wait, I'm not supposed to be laughing. This message is dealing with cancer or death or a funeral or something somber." But it is hysterically funny to picture you on a cold day in Boston, no longer in pain or paralyzed, without your pants - or endlessly chewing on your Communion Chewing Gum.

My latest writing collection is called Bury Me Naked - and in it I am finding, in the middle of Africa's suffering and poverty and dying, cause to celebrate and laugh and rejoice.

It is, I think, the laughter of Heaven. Don't you?

****

March 14, 2000
Jeremy is home for spring break and it is really nice to have him around. He is doing some of the driving for Dick's radiation appointments. Many friends have also driven him in, hopefully making the drive less lonely than it might have been. Since parking can be a problem, it is especially nice to have another person drive so that Dick doesn't have to worry about that. The radiation treatment is so short that the person who drives him can often just drive around briefly while he is having the treatment without ever bothering to actually park.

Last week Dick lost most of what was left of his thinning hair, so I shaved his head completely. Zach promptly followed suit, as did Jeremy when he got home. I think they make a mighty handsome trio. It really is a popular look these days. Several people, including me, really like the way Dick looks bald, but he finds it <u>cold</u>.

****

145

March 17, 2000
Email from Dick to his brother John in response to the question, "How are you doing?"
1) I'm down to two more treatments, one tomorrow morning (Friday) and the last one on next Monday.

2) This is a good thing, since I feel like I have the strength of a wet noodle at this point. I sleep nearly 18 hours a day. The only time I'm up for more than two or three hours is when I travel into the hospital for a treatment, taking a two to three hour nap as soon as I get back home.

It worked out well that Dad's funeral was when it was; I'm not sure I could have made it last weekend, and I know I couldn't have this weekend. Lost all my hair the week after returning. I'm surprised how much I look like Jesse Ventura. Not exactly my idol.

Looking forward greatly to the last of these treatments and getting back onto the road of healing and recovery. Time period varies from patient to patient, but it is expected that in one to two months I should be fully recovered from the radiation therapy.

****

March 27, 2000
Email "Update" from me to friends
I guess it's been a while since we sent an update. Since we VERY MUCH are aware of and appreciate your prayers and concern, I just wanted to send a note to let you know what's going on lately.

The master writer (Dick) does not really feel up to writing due to fatigue and not feeling as though he has a whole lot to say. (I am attempting to wtie this witht he new computer which has a really weeird keyboard, so I am making multil[ple mistakes and getiing quite frustrteaated .. Just want ed to hgive you a hit of wyot this would be like if I failed to proofread it.!)

Okay. Things are not BAD, just low. Dick finished the radiation on Monday 3/20. It was expected that he would feel particularly tired at the end of radiation and after because of the cumulative effects, and that is the case. He sleeps most of the day and gets up for a few hours here and there; he's generally up in the evening. He doesn't have much of an appetite since he stopped the Decadron, which is just as well, because WITH the Decadron, he was ravenous, so he gained a good bit of weight, which gave him a big belly and exacerbated his lower back (disc) problem. Whereas after the surgery and at the beginning of the radiation

146

he had lots of energy to do stuff with the computer (like setting up the web page), now he doesn't have the focus to do any significant projects.

However, last night and today he did manage to do his magic with the computer so that I am back to working on the OLD computer, which makes me happy.

Three and a half weeks ago, we got a call from Dick's mother that his father had died. Losing a parent is always difficult, but he had been in a nursing home for 8 years with advanced Alzheimer's, so his passing was in some ways a blessing. We had really said our good byes a long time ago, so the funeral was a time of celebrating his life and saying a final good bye. We were able to travel out to Syracuse for the Saturday calling hours and funeral without Dick's missing any radiation treatments. The timing was also right in that a week later, Dick would have been too fatigued to make the trip. (A week after his father died, his mother's only living sibling - her older sister - also died with Alzheimer's. We're very grateful that his mother's faith has grown so in recent months - no doubt a great help to her at this time.)

Now for the good news:

Jeremy was home for spring break the week before last. It was especially nice to have him home both so that he could spend some extra time with Dick and because he does not plan to be home for the summer. He got a job with an architecture firm in Charlottesville doing a combination of computer work with architectural plans (which he really wanted to do) and construction (which is considered to be very good experience for an architecture student.)

Zach finished the wrestling season with a 26-7 record and for the second year in a row did not get pinned. (The latter earned him the "Determination Award" at the annual banquet.) We were especially pleased that he was chosen by his peers (reportedly overwhelmingly) as next year's co-captain of the wrestling team. (It is his proud parents' contention that this has as much to do with his character as his wrestling ability.)

My latest little insight / analogy came as we were driving out to Syracuse. The New York Thruway is, to my mind, a rather dull road, but as I looked out the window at miles and miles of bare trees, it came to me: The trees aren't very attractive without their leaves - all brown and dead-looking, but when the trees are leafless, you can SEE more. Other things around them and beyond them that are not visible when there are the lovely fresh leaves, are now much easier to see. I've gotten that same sense of things through Dick's illness. It's not pretty, but other *things in life seem to come into much better focus in the "wintery" times. After the first report of cancer and all the associated treatments, life seemed to get pretty much back to "normal" for a while - the trees were covered with leaves again and looked pretty good. Then we got the news of the second cancer and my first thought - maybe I've already shared this - was that it was my fault, because I didn't learn what I was supposed to learn the first time around. I squelched that thought, because I know God doesn't work that way, but it was kind of a reminder to REMEMBER what's through the trees. There's some great stuff there.*

Well, this is kind of long - not the best way to keep in touch, but if you've stuck with me to the end, thank you! We are indeed fortunate to have you as friends.

Love,
Nancy

Chapter 19

April 26, 2000
Email from me to Ray and Jan
I still have no idea what summer plans are for us, but your comment, Ray, about joining the family for a Camp of the Woods visit got me to thinking what a HOOT that would be to have a nuclear Downing family vacation. I believe that the last time the five of us took a vacation together - just the five of us - was probably 1963 or before, since Mary Ellen was at camp for the summer before she graduated. If Mary Ellen and Mom and Dad go (and ? me and ? you) Mary Ellen says it would probably only be for two nights. Can you picture we three siblings staying in a tentel [A frame cabin] together? Even if nothing comes of this, I'm getting a kick out of imagining it!

Obviously, the reason that I am a ? for this is Dick's health. He started back on Decadron on the fourteenth because of some increasing symptoms (nausea, headaches). He also had an MRI which showed no swelling on the preliminary reading, though the ventricles were still dilated, whatever that means. The Decadron seemed to help some, so it was decreased last week, and the past couple of days he has continued to feel a little stronger, eat better, etc. I called the radiation department again today about decreasing the Decadron further, but instead of hearing back from the nurse, I got a call from the radiologist, stating that the FINAL reading of the MRI showed "a new finding" - something on the cerebellum - in the fibrous lining around the brain. . .

Bummer. Just seems like each time the poor guy starts to feel better, they find something else. He must be feeling a bit like Richard J. (for Job) Kline. God continues, however, to give encouragement. Today a coworker - after reading a note of appreciation I had given her - said that she was grateful to be working with me. And here's the good part: I can't quote her exactly - but it was something to the effect of, "You have NO IDEA what effect you have had on my spiritual life." She's someone - as are several people with whom I work - with whom I have felt free to include comments about my faith or growth - or struggles - even as I share the "facts" of this whole ordeal. Anyway, I was so touched that she would say that particular thing - not just that I'm "so strong" (she said that, too) but that I had touched the SPIRITUAL part of her life, since that's part of the WHOLE POINT of why we are here - to worship God, and part of that is to share His truth with others. I definitely do NOT have the gift of evangelism, but if our pain has allowed me to be more open about my faith, then I guess that's a good thing.

We (Zach and I) had 2 successful college visits last week - an overnight each time - to U Maine at Orono and Clarkson, in Potsdam, NY. He decided he doesn't want to go to either - wants to go south rather than north. However, after these visits, he was not yet dissuaded from the idea of mechanical engineering.

****

May 1, 2000

Today was our second "brain tumor clinic" appointment. The term sounds rather lofty to me, making me think that it is a place for answers. Once again, though, we came out with more questions than answers. One reason for the questions is that different doctors apparently "read" tests such as MRI's and CAT scans differently. This happened with an MRI of the lower back that Dick had done about three weeks ago. The preliminary report was that there were no lesions, no compression, no protrusion, and that his lower back pain was probably muscular due to previous back problems. Several years ago, he had been diagnosed with a compressed L-5 disc with spinal cord protrusion, and there was no expectation of healing. The final report of this recent MRI, done a week or two after the "preliminary" reading, indicated that there is, in fact, compression of the disc, but no protrusion. So the same "picture" did not look the same to everyone who saw it. There is a similar situation now with a body CAT scan that was done in February and reported as fine, but now interpreted as showing a mass in Dick's pelvis. That's a big difference in interpretation, and very confusing and frustrating for me!

****

May 4, 2000

Email from me to Ray and Jan

It's been a tough week. The brain tumor clinic was full of surprises on Monday - first the mention of the MASS in front of the lumbar / sacral spine. I was dumbfounded by this, no one having mentioned it before, and this doc sort of stating it "by the way." Anyway, I think it was really the use of the term MASS that got me. In fact, the oncologist HAD mentioned that there was "something" there, but he felt it was consistent with Dick's having had surgery and radiation and several complications there. When I spoke to him Tuesday, he reiterated this, saying that the only ways to tell if it was tumor vs. other "something" would be biopsy or repeat CAT scans to see if it has grown. Dick has a CAT scan scheduled for tomorrow, and we're scheduled to see the oncologist next Wednesday, presumably to discuss the findings and future plans.

Meanwhile, there are the three (yes three) new spots (presumably tumors) in the brain to consider. Unfortunately, they are not localized to one spot, leading the doctors to believe that there might be cancer cells in the cerebrospinal fluid, which is floating around the brain and seeding new tumors. Dick had a spinal tap yesterday, the results of which should be back tomorrow. If the fluid is positive for cancer cells, we'll have to "reconsider" what to do next (? brain chemo?). If it is negative, he will proceed with the stereotactic radiosurgery, which is scheduled for Monday May 8. He's already had a "fusion MRI" done for that (we went into Boston for a 10PM appointment for that last night - unbelievable, huh?) If it is a go for that (the radiosurgery), we'll go in at 7:00 Monday AM for him to be surgically fitted with a metal crown and have a CAT scan. The CAT scan will then be put together with the MRI and computerized to plan the radiation. He would end up getting more radiation from that one day than the 4 weeks of daily radiation combined.

Obviously, any way we look at this - it's not a real pretty picture. Obviously, we'd rather there not be cancer cells in the CSF, and the prospect of brain chemo is unpleasant at best. However, even the "best case" scenario at this point looks a bit rough, with even more radiation. And then there's that MASS. Right now we have a couple of days of waiting for more data, so that leaves a little larger window of hope, but while I don't want to be pessimistic, unwarranted optimism is not helpful either. The bottom line remains the same: "For your ways are not My ways, neither are your thoughts My thoughts, says the Lord God Almighty. For as the heavens are higher than the earth, so are My thoughts higher than your thoughts, and My ways than your ways." (Quoted from memory, so it may not be exact, but as I recall, that's the gist of it.) I can't believe this is all happening, but it IS. I truly have no doubt that even at this point, God is completely capable of healing Dick, but I also know that He may or may not choose to do so, and either way - though I don't understand it - I know that He loves Dick and me and Jeremy and Zach even more than we love each other. And - corny as that old song sounds - it is true that, "I don't know what the future holds, but I know Who holds the future." I'm grateful for these solid truths now,

because when I get into the emotional realm, it's a heck of a lot more shaky.
We are ever grateful for prayers and loving concern.

****

.

May 6, 2000
Email from Dick to friends (36 on the list now)
Title: "Silence Broken"

It has been quite awhile since I have written a general update to you all. Nancy wrote one on March 27 and indicted that I was feeling pretty fatigued and not really up to much of anything other than sleeping most of the day.

I finished radiation on 3/20. The first two weeks went with no serious side effects whatsoever. The last two weeks were a different story. I started to have trouble breathing (they were able to give me an inhaler which helped), and weariness and fatigue settled in until it just became impossible to do much of anything other than lay around the house and moan "woe is me" :-<   During the next four weeks (after radiation stopped) the fatigue got somewhat worse instead of better.

During this time in my life I had two constants: I was able to arrange my sleep schedule such that I was able to go to church on Sunday morning and to attend the weekly Bible study which conveniently meets in our home on Tuesday evenings. Outside of those two weekly events, everything else was planned on a last minute basis, if I was feeling up to it. And indeed, several fun times with friends were squeezed in at various times. Thanks for being flexible with us.

The good news is that about two weeks ago I started to feel somewhat better. The cough and the fatigue are lessening (although still with me). Each day I usually feel a little bit stronger than the day before. A positive sign to be headed in a positive direction.

Unfortunately, not all of the recent news is good. I have recently had more tests, and not all the results are favorable. In particular, a recent two month post-op brain scan (MRI) has shown another three new tumors in the brain, all small, but there nonetheless. The preferred method for removing these tumors is stereotactic radiosurgery, a technique where they use a very high dosage of radiation that is highly focused on the tumor, thereby burning the tumor tissue. This technique is available in only a few places in the world at the present time. I was scheduled to have this procedure performed this coming Monday (May

152

8). *However, this was contingent upon the results of a test that I had last Wednesday.*

The worry was that the three present tumors are scattered throughout the brain (i.e., not localized to one area). One possible explanation could be that there are cancer cells floating in the spinal fluid which circulates through the brain and the spinal cord. On Wednesday I had a spinal tap to draw off some of the spinal fluid for analysis. Unfortunately, we found out Friday that the spinal fluid tested positive; there are abnormal cells in the fluid. Because of this, the stereotactic radiosurgery for Monday has been postponed and at present we don't know what the course of treatment will be.

All this is complicated further by the fact that some of my doctors (I'm seeing four specialists at present) are concerned about a "mass" at the base of my spine (in the pelvic region) and of course there is the abnormal vertebra in my neck that still needs to be checked out since the last round of radiation. I have further tests scheduled for this week (to check out the neck) and doctors appointments to discuss the situation and treatment options.

Obviously, the situation is pretty serious, though not completely hopeless. Please be praying that Nancy and I, and Jeremy and Zachary would continue to feel a sense of peace as we rest in God's hands. To tell the truth, there have been several times in the past couple of months that I haven't "felt" God's loving presence, even though I know He is there.

****

May 7, 2000

Friday night I decided to stay home with Dick instead of going out to a youth praise event. Zach was not home, but Dick and I had a very pleasant time together. He grilled hamburgers for himself and Portobello mushrooms for me, and we feasted out on the deck. The air temperature was perfect: no wind, not hot, not cool. Perfect. We talked, agreeing to be completely open with each other, sharing our most morbid thoughts as well as our positive ones. Better to get them out in the open, we decided, rather than letting them smolder inside. My morbid (selfish) thoughts related to my fear that Dick will die. If he does die in the next couple of years, that will mean that he leaves me at about the same time that Zach goes to college, and I will be all alone. Ouch. His most morbid thought was that he won't be around a year from now - not a pre-monition, mind you - just a thought.

I also mentioned my concerns about his desire to be cremated. That's fine with me, but what do I do with the ashes? I certainly can't leave them on the mantle - I'd be sure to knock them over - and if Jeremy, Zach and I decide to take a hike in the White Mountains to scatter them there, I'll probably do something dumb like scatter them on bear poop or something, and then do something totally inappropriate like laughing! Dick said if it was just the three of us, it would be okay. He said "it would be like it often is, with me being the only one not laughing!" He suggested that we could just scatter the ashes in the woods next to the house, but not tell the neighbors. (We could just tell them we have the feeling that Dick is still with us - "all around us" . . .)

So much for the morbid thoughts. He also said today that he was becoming more open to the idea of a complete miracle - that maybe when the doctors have said that there is no more that they can do - that God might choose to completely eliminate the cancer. I am completely convinced that this is possible, but it is not what I am expecting. It is a difficult balance: to have faith that God can heal, but not to presume that He will. I believe He loves us more than we love ourselves and more than we love each other, but I also believe that His thoughts and ways are not ours; His are higher.

Yesterday Dick finally wrote an email to our friends. He hadn't written since the end of February, shortly after his surgery. He was quite fatigued from the radiation and really had no energy to write or anything to say, for that matter. We talked a week or two ago about that. I think because people have been so very supportive and have given us such positive responses to the emails (saying how our faith and strength has encouraged them), we have put a little pressure on ourselves to be sure that we send positive messages - not that the news is always positive, but we have been somewhat careful to reflect a positive, faith-filled attitude.

Despite the fact that our faith remains firm, the feelings have not always been positive in the last month or so. I suggested that Dick should feel free to write that. His email did mention his not "feeling" God's presence sometimes, and already, in the last two days, we have received some very warm and thoughtful responses to that.

Yesterday I was talking to our neighbor, whose mother has been very ill for about five months. He and his sister have chosen, following a rather lengthy hospitalization for the mother, to care for her at home. It is a full-time job, overwhelming at times as well as confining. When I mentioned how supportive our friends have been during Dick's illness, our neighbor was pleased for us, but indicated that he has not felt the same support from his friends. He feels that some of them have backed off - not reaching out to him as he would have liked and hoped. I suggested that he might need to let them know how he feels. So many of our friends have expressed appreciation that we are sharing our lives with them - the ups and downs - and the outpouring of love that we have received from that little (selfish?) effort on our part has been unbelievable. People who live at a distance have written thoughtful emails and sent cards and notes. People who are close have responded by bringing us flowers or food.

Here are some more encouraging emails we have received, in response to Dick's "Silence Broken" one.
From Dick's cousin Terry:
Thanks for the update. The whole situation stinks and you don't deserve to be going through all of this. I know there is a greater plan....but this still stinks! We continue to think of you and pray for all of you. If we can do anything......please don't hesitate. Dick, maybe I should never have introduced you to fooling around with radios and stuff when you were small.....maybe you did too many experiments with all those old vacuum tube radios! Oh God - just get better.

From Anne:
Your news is of course in human terms quite overwhelming. But YOU, in your witness over these last months and months have made US strong. I (emphasized) will carry YOUR news that God is good and absolutely trustworthy, and has mercies that are new every morning. Satan does not like it that you, and we, believe this of God. That this precious family which has suffered so much still loves and trusts and leans on Him. The war is on. Dick, Hudson Taylor once said, when he was asked if he was always conscious of abiding with Christ: "While sleeping last night did I cease to abide in your house because I was unconscious of the fact? We should never be conscious of NOT abiding in Christ..." (p 444, volume 2)
And one of my favorite verses is in John 10, "No one shall snatch them out of His hand," said Jesus.
We LOVE you!!!! Great is HIS faithfulness.

From Dave (Dick's best man):
 . . . *I want to tell you that your life is completely in God's hands. It is He who made you. He gives you each breath. He controls each cell in your body. He is using this illness for his glory - you have already testified to that. In your suffering you more fully understand Christ's suffering and sacrifice for us. Your hope now is not in your own strength or medical techniques - though these are part of the present plan. Your hope is in God. Regardless of what details the future holds, you will live forever. I pray that God will spare your physical life for many more years, and I rejoice that He is watching over you every moment in a perfect way. Do not give up believing.*

From Bob:
 Thank you for the latest email giving us all the latest news on your condition. I know I speak for a lot of us, that we want to know so we can pray more specifically - whether you currently have good news or bad news. Barb and I have been praying for all of you a lot these weeks and months.
 I can't quite imagine the emotional drain that this long ordeal has put all of you through. I was glad to hear that thus far you have been able to go to church and attend the Bible study in your home. That's great. Dick, you spoke about not always "feeling God's loving presence." I'm not surprised. It's at times like this that the rest of us - that don't have to go through the emotional and physical strain that you do - can be faithful in our prayers for you and claim the truth of God's love even though you may not feel it. Dick, Barb and I want you to know how much we love and care for you and Nancy and Zach and Jeremy. We will keep you in our prayers.

From Kathy (close friend since Jeremy was born):
 ...I'm trying to get into the habit of looking at the present from the perspective of the future, when all will be clear, and the crises of today will assume their rightful place on the list of "what really matters". But, as Dick said, sometimes we easily feel God's presence, and sometimes it's a lot harder. And that's when friends and their prayers really matter, to carry us (me) over those times of not understanding the plan. I know your faith is strong. My hope is that on the darker days, when it's hard to fathom what the purpose in all this must be, that the prayers of all of your friends will carry you along until you feel stronger again. Thank God for friends. You guys have been such good friends to so many people. I

hope it's all returning to you now, multiplied several times over! As you asked, our prayer will be that you all feel peaceful with whatever lies ahead for you, and that you will continue to see God's blessings in the midst of this terrible situation your family is facing. Our love to you - thanks for keeping us on your list, and letting us know how you're doing.

Chapter 20

May 10, 2000

In the midst of running back and forth to the hospital and dealing with brain tumors and other very big issues, life goes on. Work has been very busy for me; visits to my office have been about fifty per day in addition to the over forty daily medicines I give. I suppose the bright part of that is that I am not left with a lot of time to worry.

Last week was the National Honor Society induction for Zach - a very good thing. It was good to have something positive for Zach, since he has had to deal with several disappointments in his life lately in addition to his dad having cancer. However, he is very resilient, and his faith is strong. I got a glimpse of that last night when he showed me the day's devotional from a booklet he has been following. The story was about a battle in 1346 in which King Edward had put his son, the prince, in charge of the battle, while the King waited off to the side in case he was needed. After a bit, the prince decided that he really needed his dad, so he called for help. King Edward didn't come, instead responding, "Go tell my son that I am not so inexperienced a commander as not to know when help is needed, nor so careless a father as to not send it." The point that we both got from the story was that sometimes it seems as though God is not answering our prayers, but He knows exactly what we need. I was glad that Zach showed me that - both because it was very timely, and also because it showed me where his thoughts are.

****

May 11, 2000

When we saw Dr. Huberman yesterday, we discussed pain medication. Dick had had severe pain the previous night - in his upper back, shoulders and neck. Dr. Huberman feels that pain control is very important, so he wrote a new prescription for a long acting pain medicine (Oxycontin) and another one for "breakthrough pain" (Roxycodone). He assures me that it is not harmful for Dick to take this as needed; constipation is the one anticipated side effect, and that is just not a problem for Dick! I also asked Dr. Huberman about the possibility of Dick's taking amytriptyline (Elavil), which I had heard is good for chronic pain. Since it is a tricyclic antidepressant, I figured that Dick could take

care of two things (pain and depression) with one pill, and without some of the side effects that Paxil has, but Dr. Huberman said that he would still need pain medicine even with the Elavil, so it would be best to not change anything now. (I was pleased that he did not think it was a stupid question.)

****

May 12, 2000
Email from Dick to friends
Title: "Good news?"
Thursday:

I want to thank everyone for praying for us. Your prayers have already been answered (although there is still a lot to pray for). I saw my oncologist Wednesday, to discuss my overall situation and the results of my most recent tests (CAT scan of pelvic region). Compared to all the bad news we have received in the past several weeks, things look much more hopeful.

I'll run through the issues one at a time, starting with the good news and then continuing on to the things which are still unknown and / or of concern.

First is the "mass" at the base of the spine. This was first pointed out to us by the neuro-oncologist last week and was presented as a probable new cancer site. However, I had a CAT scan performed last week and was told yesterday by my "body" oncologist that the CAT scan shows the mass to be the same size as it was in the February CAT scan, and furthermore, the February scan shows it to be the same size as a CAT scan taken last July. This means that whatever this mass is, it is not growing (i.e., not an active cancer) and that the most likely scenario is that it is just scar tissue, or something similar, from the many surgeries I have had in the pelvic region. This is great news since it means that "the mass" can be crossed off the list of things that need to be scheduled for treatment.

You may recall that since January, there was the issue of the possible tumor in my C-4 vertebra in my neck (remember the "Heavens are telling the glory of God, or don't leave home without your pants" email?) When I had the whole brain radiation treatments, they opened the field of radiation to also include the neck. Wednesday night I had an MRI of the neck region which will be compared to the one taken in

January to see if things look better, the same, or worse. We will probably find out Friday the results of this scan.
Friday:
We received a preliminary report this afternoon; basically the neck appears to have no change. I guess the neck just continues to be something to monitor. At present, there is no need to perform any treatments in this area.
This brings us to the last two problem areas which are the spinal fluid and the three new brain tumors. Recall that the brain tumors could be treated by stereotactic radiosurgery (highly focused beams of radiation), but not if the spinal fluid contained cancerous cells. Recall that the spinal fluid showed abnormal cells. There appears to be a difference of opinion on the most likely conclusion. My regular oncologist doesn't necessarily think they are cancerous because:
1) my spinal fluid chemistry (protein, sugar level, etc.) is normal, and usually, but not always, the spinal fluid chemistry is off from its regular levels when infected with cancer cells.
2) also, colon cancer rarely spreads to the spinal fluid. My oncologist has never seen a case where this has happened (20+ years?), although he has read about such cases in the literature.
It is clear that my neuro-oncologist thinks otherwise. Thus the canceling of treating the three brain tumors with the stereotactic radiosurgery at this time.
The present plan is to wait for another 5 to 6 weeks and to repeat the brain scan (MRI) and spinal tap at that time to look for changes in any of the above, and then treat appropriately. Meanwhile, I'm to try to rest up and to hopefully fully recover from the fatigue/cough from the brain radiation received in March.
Things to pray for:
1) That the spinal fluid does not contain cancer cells. The fact that my oncologist said that colon cancer spreading to the spinal fluid is extremely rare is a double edged sword. The flip side is that if the colon cancer has spread to the spinal fluid, there are no known protocols for treatment. We'll get one chance using an experimental chemo of some sort.
2) Pray that the next 5 to 6 weeks will go quickly and peacefully without complications.
3) Pray for my complete recovery from the brain radiation.

****

NANCY KLINE

May 12, 2000
Email from Don to Dick:
Thanks for the update. Sorry to learn that the battle continues on so many fronts. You remain in our constant prayers.

When I think of you, I still see a party - a joyous celebration. It takes place in your back yard. You and Nancy are standing on the deck you and Zach built and all your friends are gathered in the yard. It is very packed. You tell your story - there is not a dry eye "in-the-house". Then the joyous celebration of God's healing begins. We are all drunk with the holy spirit offering praise and song to our Lord for His mighty work in your life - your healing. Your story and the party are both a great witness and blessing. It fits with your current situation - you only have a great celebration when the healing by our Lord has been miraculous!

So how about hastening this celebration along? I was listening to the radio last week and they were telling the story of Elisha (I think; my mind was in different places) healing the boy. He put his body over the boy and he had to go back and pray for him more than once. The point being - touch is important and to keep praying until you see results!

Thus, if you haven't already done it, why not an all day / weekend prayer vigil for Dick? People could sign up - say teams of five on the hour. Dick, you could even nap during some of the prayers. Start at nine in the morning and have hourly slots all day / weekend.

I would be happy to help coordinate an effort such as this via e-mail and the phone.

****

May 17, 2000
Lots of anger this morning - in my head and spilling out on my face as I took my early morning walk. So much is not <u>right</u> now: the picture doesn't look good for Dick (I think the neuro oncologist thinks cancer is in the spinal fluid); bad pain in Dick's neck continues - (why?); constant headache; little appetite. Our church is falling apart; the elders all resigned and a couple of them left the church - one after 42 years there. Thor (Jeremy's cat who is living with us for a year) is not making a great adjustment to life in Walpole - he's a wild cat. Both boys cars are having trouble, etc, etc...

I started to make a ledger - list the bad first and get that out of the way - and then focus on the good things in our lives. But what if the good isn't as long - or doesn't <u>seem</u> as long? What does that song say?

161

"Take my heart and form it; take my mind, transform it; take my will, CONFORM IT TO YOURS, oh, Lord."

The day stayed sad for me. I cried when I read a letter from one of the teachers at school saying he was going to do a bike ride in support of cancer research. He offered to wear on his shirt the names of "loved ones" who have cancer. I cried more when Marcia stopped in to see me, and then later when I went to visit Arlene. I was so sad for Dick. Why couldn't he either have a good prognosis or feel good - at least one of the two?

****

May 18, 2000
Dick responded to Don's suggestion:

I have been thinking about your prayer suggestion. It sounds great to Nancy and me. There are several reasons why we don't feel like "we" can coordinate this; it just wouldn't feel right, plus health issues really limit our day to day capabilities.

Maybe we could dedicate a Saturday, hopefully sometime soon. Some people could come to the house for laying on hands, and others who are too far away to travel could pick an hour to be praying at the same time. Maybe 7 one hour slots, 9-10, 10-11,..., 4-5. Please contact Nancy to discuss which Saturday.

... Let me know your most recent thoughts and if you are willing to coordinate. It's OK if you can't. My health is not good and my physical condition seems to be deteriorating somewhat this week. I believe time is of the essence.

****

May 21, 2000

We received a copy of the email that Don sent to everyone on our prayer list stating that there would be a day of prayer here for Dick on June 3. It invited people to come for one of three pre-determined hours or to pray wherever they were that day. Don suggested that people notify either Carolyn or Noel (our associate pastor) to indicate when they would be praying. There was also a sign up sheet at church this morning. What a nice gesture - for people to be willing to join on a specific day just to pray for Dick!

****

May 24, 2000

Well, it has been a busy, rough few days. Last week on Wednesday, the neuro-oncologist started Dick on a low dose of Nortriptyline (a tricyclic antidepressant) for headache control. On Thursday, Dr. Huberman increased Dick's long-acting pain medicine. Jeremy and Liz, who had both been here for about a week, left Friday for Virginia, where they plan to live and work for the summer. Dick felt a little better on Saturday and Sunday, but then there was Monday night - the night before last.

I awoke at 2:15 AM to find Dick kneeling with his head on the floor in the bathroom - unable to get up. He crawled back to bed, then collapsed before he could get up on the bed. We finally managed to get him up, but sleep did not return for me after that. Dick twitched all night - the kind of twitching one does when falling asleep - and I wondered if he was going to have a seizure. Seizures were listed in my nurses' Drug Handbook under "common life-threatening side effects" for Nortriptyline. Also listed, as non life-threatening side effects, were drowsiness, dizziness, and ringing in the ears - all things which Dick had experienced during the day on Monday. Perhaps foolishly (hindsight is always clearer...) we had decided that he should take the Monday night dose of the medication, thinking the side effects might diminish as he grew more accustomed to the drug; and it was helping his headache.

At 5:15 AM, Dick sat up rather quickly, saying that he had to urinate. I jumped up and sat on his right, urging him to take it slowly, but before he could even attempt to get up, he flopped over to the right onto me. I helped him back to his left side, and after a couple of minutes, I asked if he still had to go to the bathroom. "I already went," he replied. I thought he might have wet himself, but he hadn't; he just thought he had gotten up and gone to the bathroom.

Just after that he developed an excruciating headache, which brought him to tears. I brought him the short-acting pain medicine, and within fifteen minutes, he was feeling better. Meanwhile, it was clear that I would not be going to work, and I didn't know if Dick would need to go to the hospital, so at about 5:30 I called Cathy, the head school nurse, to arrange for a substitute for me.

I supposed that I would need help if Dick needed to go into Boston to the doctor's office (which would not open until eight or nine o'clock) or to the hospital, so I called Carolyn's husband at about 7:30 to see if he might be available later if needed. He said that he would be. I had also called Bobbie (sometimes I am especially grateful to know early risers!) to ask for hints for getting Dick up slowly to avoid what I assumed was a significant blood pressure drop. I hadn't checked it; I guess I didn't really want to know what it was.

Bobbie promptly suggested that Dick might be dehydrated and recommended that I give him Gatorade, which I did not have. She offered to get some and bring it to us, and I accepted her offer. She brought that, checked Dick's blood pressure, went to work for a meeting for an hour, then returned to spend the whole day with us. What a wonderful support that was! She is a good friend, and she is also a very good nurse. I wonder if I would have taken the day off work in a similar situation.

As often happens in crisis situations, Dick's doctors were both away, but I spoke with the neurology nurse, Loretta, and she agreed with Bobbie and me that his problems were probably from the Nortriptyline and significant dehydration. Bobbie and I strongly encouraged Dick to drink. He really hates to drink, so this was not easy for him. However, according to the doctor who was covering for Dr. Huberman, his only other option was to go to the hospital for IV fluids, so Dick really put forth a concerted effort to imbibe freely of Gatorade.

Meanwhile, Tom and Carolyn had come bearing yet more Gatorade and a "husband" - one of those things with a back and arms that one puts on a bed against a wall, for the purpose of sitting up in bed. They also carried one of the stuffed chairs from the living room up to our bedroom, and by 5:00, Dick was able to sit up in that. What wonderful friends we have!

For supper, we set up a card table in the bedroom for Zach, Dick and me to eat together. Zach thoughtfully put a tablecloth and candle on the table so that we could eat in the style to which we were accustomed.

One of the most amazing things about the day was a story that Carolyn told us last evening about Tara, one of the young adults with whom Dick had worked in a Bible study. Tara had been driving to work yesterday when she felt a great urge to fast for Dick. She was moved to tears as she was driving and called Carolyn when she got to work to ask if there was anything going on with Dick. Now that is no coincidence! Tara was concerned enough to pray and fast for us without knowing anything of the crisis that Dick was experiencing. Certainly God heard and answered those prayers, because the peace I felt throughout the day was fairly extraordinary. I did not feel overwhelmed - just tremendously supported. I even felt hopeful about Dick's physical status - hopeful that the fluids would really help, and they did.

Today Mary Ellen came to stay with Dick because I was uneasy about leaving him alone. He hadn't seemed to have good judgment about getting up slowly yesterday. When he was lying down, he would feel great and then think he could just jump right up, forgetting that quick changes of position caused him to feel extremely shaky and weak. How nice to have a sister who would come at a moment's notice (and it helped that she is a nurse, too) to give me the peace of mind I needed to go to work. Dick actually did much better during the day, even going downstairs several times before the day was over.

I thought we were over the rough part, but at 10:15 PM (now) he got up to go to the bathroom - weak and shaky again - and with a headache. Today's relief didn't last long. What now? He has already had the long-acting and the short-acting pain medicines; he hasn't had the Nortriptyline in 48 hours, and he is doing well with drinking. I am fresh out of ideas of what to do next. I <u>really</u> hate crises in the dark! Does it have to be this way? Do I have to complain and worry? I've just seen God's amazing grace for the past 48 hours and here I am, anxious about the next eight hours. I just feel so alone! There are people who have said that I could call at night (including Debbie and Bob next door), but in a half-stupor myself at night, it's hard to know when I need to call someone or when I should just ride it out. I'm thinking of part of a song I really like by Caedmon's Call, and to me it is a prayer: ". . .You knew this day long before you made me out of dirt. And You know the plans that You have for me; and You can't plan the ends and not plan the means; and so I suppose I just need some peace to get me to sleep."

****

May 24, 2000
Email from Dick to friends
Title: "A specific prayer request"
I have a very specific prayer request. I'm going in for a repeat spinal tap this Friday morning. The first one, performed about 6 weeks ago showed "abnormal cells" in the fluid, but the pathologist did not declare them to be cancer cells in the final report. It is important what the outcome of this test is. In particular, it is important that there is not cancer in the spinal fluid because there are not any known protocols (treatments) for colon cancer which has spread to the spinal fluid; it is a

very rare event, and therefore no significant trials have been attempted or reported.

As always, we rest in God's hands, but it would be very good news (a miracle ?) to receive a report that the spinal fluid is clear! We should hear the results sometime next week. I'll send out a list of other specific prayer request sometime before the June 3 prayer date. God bless.

****

May 27, 2000
Email from Dick to friends (42 now)
Title: "June 3 - Day of Prayer for Dick Kline"
This is a follow up message to the one from Don Coffin (who is organizing this event along with Carolyn Churchill). Don is on a week's vacation, so that is why this message is from me instead of Don.

Please note that the prayer times at our house have changed to allow an evening prayer hour for those that want to come to the house but have to work during the day. The new times are the following:

10 a.m. (same as before)
1 p.m. (same as before)
8 p.m. (new evening hour)
The former 2 p.m. time slot has been canceled. Hopefully this won't exclude anyone, but I will need to conserve my energy on that day and this seemed the best way to address other people's schedules. Thanks for your understanding.

The following is a list of specific prayer requests both for now and for that day:

1) I had the repeat spinal tap on Friday morning (May 26). Everything went well during the procedure. We probably will not hear the results until later next week. Be praying that God performs a miracle and that the spinal fluid is clear (cancer free).

2) I am scheduled for a repeat brain scan on June 19th. Pray that the three "tumors" have not grown significantly, or multiplied in number, and are still small enough to be treatable by the stereotactic radiosurgery.

3) Pray for a second miracle, that the three tumors no longer exist!

4) Continue to pray for Jeremy in Virginia this summer. We believe he is in the right place, but it is difficult being away from his Dad and family at this time.

166

5) *Continue to pray for Zachary (a senior in high school next year) as so much is going on in his life (choosing a vocation, college, etc.) at the same time that life at home is often interrupted, sometimes in the middle of the night, by a new medical crisis. Pray that he would be able to visit the colleges in which he is currently most interested.*

6) *Pray for Nancy, who has to be at least three people at once. She is the only gainfully employed member of the family, has to do all of her housework (laundry, cooking, cleaning, etc.), has to do all my work (dishes, mowing lawn, etc.), has to be my nearly full time nurse (24 hours per day). She's doing a great job at all this, but I don't know how she manages at times. A little prayer support goes a long way.*

The following are additional prayer requests from Nancy:

7) *Pray for the neck - the current source of pain. The last MRI showed more bone involvement. This is assumed to be cancer, though it has never been biopsied. Pray that it would get better - cancer or not!*

8) *Pray for a limit on the crises in the middle of the night. Crises in the dark are tough for Nancy.*

9) *Pray that we might be able to have a mini family vacation at the Cape on Father's Day weekend. With the boys growing and gone for the summer, we're looking for quality rather than quantity time together.*

10) *Pray that we would continue to want God's will more than any of the above.*

I'll send out more requests when I think of them. This is a start.

God bless you.

****

May 28, 2000

I still wake up each time Dick gets up to go to the bathroom, and I go with him if there is any unsteadiness, so I do not get any uninterrupted nights of sleep any more, but at least Dick is feeling considerably better than he was a few days ago. The night after Mary Ellen came to stay with him was not too bad, but the next morning he was still shaky, so I didn't want to leave him home alone. After taking my morning walk, I called Mary Ellen to ask her come to stay with him again. I also called to tell the people at work that I would be in late; I wanted to stay with Dick while he showered and changed his ileostomy bag, knowing that Mary Ellen would not arrive for over an hour. In fact, Dick seemed much stronger and did not seem to need help, so I told Mary Ellen that she did not need to come, and I went to work at around 9:00.

The folks at work continue to be <u>most</u> understanding and supportive, putting up with my late arrivals and early departures.

To my great surprise, at around 11:30, Dick appeared at my office, bearing six long-stemmed roses in celebration of our twenty-fourth anniversary, which is tomorrow. I told him he was making me look bad, because I had told people that I was late because he was sick; but of course I was thrilled to see him - as was everyone else.

Gentle Breeze:

May 2000 - June 2000

Chapter 21

May 31, 2000
Email from Dick to (48) friends and relatives
Title: "The first miracle"

Recall that last week I sent out 10 specific prayer requests. The first one was the following:

"1) I had the repeat spinal tap on Friday morning (May 26). Everything went well during the procedure. We probably will not hear the results until later next week. Be praying that God performs a miracle and that the spinal fluid is clear (cancer free)."

This prayer request was probably the most important since there are no known treatments for colon cancer that has metastasized to the spinal fluid (i.e., my condition would have been considered terminal and the only available treatment would have been some unproven experimental chemotherapy that the docs cooked up in the back room).

One of my doctors called this afternoon with the results of the spinal tap. Nancy and I have coined the name "doctor doom and gloom" ever since the first spinal tap which had "suspicious / abnormal" cells in the fluid. At that point the doctor canceled the previously planned stereotactic radiosurgery for the three tumors in the brain, because he said there would be no point in treating these tumors if the spinal fluid was infected with the colon cancer.

Dr. doom and gloom called this afternoon to say that the spinal fluid is clear, there are no abnormal, suspicious, or cancerous cells in the fluid. The fluid is CLEAR! He also said he would be contacting the other two docs (the neurosurgeon and the neuro-radiologist; these are the two that would perform the stereotactic radiosurgery) to discuss the next steps.

This is the miracle that we were hoping for. God is good!

Remember my next two requests:

"2) I am scheduled for a repeat brain scan on June 19th. Pray that the three "tumors" have not grown significantly, or multiplied in number, and are still small enough to be treatable by the stereotactic radiosurgery.

3) Pray for a second miracle, that the three tumors no longer exist!"

Nancy and I are rejoicing greatly tonight. Thanks for your prayers and we are looking forward to this Saturday. God bless.

****

June 3, 2000
What an amazing day - the Day of Prayer for Dick and his family. There were people all over the US as well as some in England and Africa who had agreed to pray for us on this day. What a gift! The three hours when people actually gathered here to pray were indeed special. We really agreed in prayer: bold prayers for healing, but with acknowledgment that this might not be God's will, and prayers of praise for His love and redemption. Twice Dick was anointed with oil. At 10:00, there were eight people here praying together; two of those people we had never met before! At 1:00 there were eleven of us; and at 8:00, twenty-seven of us gathered in the family room to pray! In addition to the people who came, Carolyn had compiled a list of about 50 people who were not here, but had contacted her to say that they would be praying at different specified times during the day.

Carolyn had also asked the young adults, for whom she and Dick had led a Bible study, to write her notes saying how Dick and I had affected their lives. One from Tara was especially kind. She said some nice things about me and then this about Dick: "What amazes me about Dick is that in the most difficult time of his life, he still has the ability to encourage, uplift and bless every person he comes in contact with. Through thick and thin, whether there were twenty people at Bible study or one, he was there - being committed when there was no commitment. Above all these things, I long to have an understanding of the Word of God as Dick does, and to be able to share it with others as clearly as he does. Thank you, Dick." This message was from Kerri: "Dick has shown me that perseverance in prayer is key when faced with trials in life. Love is greater than anything. God has more in store for us than we have ever imagined, and no matter what circumstances you are in in life, God will always use you if you allow him to. Tell him thank you for being a great example."

****

June 3, 2000
Email from Dick to friends
Title: "Thanks for the day of prayer"
Yesterday was quite a day. Even if I were to write several hundred words, it wouldn't begin to express the gratitude for such an outpouring

171

of love. Thanks to you all. The three times at the home were wonderful times of prayer and anointing. And we had a long list on the table in the room of others who couldn't make it to the house, but were praying for us at specific times throughout the entire day.

Thank you.

Thank you, Thank you.

I'm sure I will write more later.

God bless, and love to you all.

****

June 4, 2000

We had many responses today from people who were involved in prayer, from near and far.

From Bob:

...Dick, if it wasn't perfectly clear to you before yesterday, I trust it is now that you and Nancy have had a huge impact on people... You are both more of the "behind-the-scenes" type of people rather than the "up-front-give-a-speech" type of people. But don't minimize the impact you have had. Your quiet faithfulness behind the scenes has been deeply felt and very clearly noted by all those around you. Your character is impeccable, and you put your beliefs into action. It's impossible to overlook that kind of sincere testimony to the grace of God.

Dick, you are deeply loved and highly respected. All of your friends are praying for you as you battle this cancer. I trust we shall have many times of great rejoicing in the weeks and months ahead as we see God's answers to our many prayers.

We continue to pray for you. This morning in church you were in my mind almost through the entire service. I found myself praying for you at many points in the worship service this morning. We'll keep it up.

I love you, Dick. Thank you for being such a good friend.

From Sandy, one of the youth leaders at our church:

...I love your web page and the desire you have to keep everyone informed of your progress in your battle. I hope you both were as blessed as I was by the outpouring of people praying for you this past weekend. God is so good and He has blessed so many people with your

friendship and love. May your family be enjoying this time of encouragement. I hope we see Dick becoming perkier every day. I love using the word perky in describing you as it really does not fit well but the current situation makes it such a fun word to use in describing your being more active and involved in the art of living under the cloud of cancer.

****

June 5, 2000
Email from Dick to friends
Title: "Satan is not happy today."

I know that Satan is a bit of a controversial character in theology these days, some people thinking that he is alive and "well" and others not able to believe that God would allow such an absolute embodiment of evil to exist at all.

It became obvious to Nancy and me Sunday and even stronger since today, (actually, last night during difficult times), that Satan is not happy about all the prayers that were lifted up for us this past Saturday.

As those of you who saw me Saturday know, it was clear that God granted a special time of Grace Saturday in that I was in peak physical shape (for my condition) and able to fully partake in the times of prayer and even times of fellowship afterwards.

However, it is clear to us now that God is allowing Satan to touch my body once again, and that with it returns a lot of pain and nausea, and lack of sleep, and run away emotions. Please be praying for us that the pain and nausea will subside. It just happens that Nancy and I have an appointment with my main oncologist this afternoon in Boston. Maybe a change in medications will help?

Thanks for your prayers, and God bless you all.

P.S. - I believe that everyone on this email prayer list is on it because at some point over the past two and one half years you requested to be added. If the updates / requests ever become too frequent and you feel like this is just one more source of SPAM, then just send me a short email asking to have your name removed. There will be no hard feelings, so don't hesitate, and of course, you could always get information from the web site which I do update from time to time.

****

We got some quick responses today to that email, including many assuring Dick that they are glad to be on the email list.
From Nadjia:
Hold on. And if you can't, just let God hold onto you. The 23rd Psalm has always been a comfort to me. Recently I heard a commentary about the phrase, "He leadeth me beside the still waters," which I had never considered. Sheep, being the wooly creatures that they are, are terrified of water. Should they slip in, the weight of their wet bodies and the lack of strength in their weak legs, would surely cause them to drown. The shepherd leads them carefully BESIDE the water. Without the shepherd, in such a fatally precarious place, the sheep might either die of thirst or drown. As the sheep must trust the shepherd, I'm learning that in the most serious and anxiety ridden circumstances, I must remember that HE WILL LEAD ME BESIDE THE STILL WATERS. May you sense your good Shepherd with you. My prayers are with you.

From Carolyn:
Well Satan isn't going to win and he can't keep us from praying, so that's what we'll do.
Also a little happy note...
I was emailing Kelly and giving her your updates, prayer requests and info on the prayer time for last Sat. Well I found out the address I was sending all this to was wrong, by one letter. I received a note from this girl and she wanted to know how I knew her. I explained that I made a mistake on the address and was sorry. She just emailed me back saying that was okay because she is a Christian and was praying for all these things anyway. So is GOD good or what???

From our good friend Jim:
Your email prompts a brief response from me before I go off to work this morning, in the way of a short story. Sunday afternoon (after seeing you Saturday night) the kids had a piano recital, and then we went to our friends' house for a meal with some others. The kids were all playing outside and (as you might expect) I was on one of the teams for "capture the flag." These friends have a very big and very black cat, more panther than house cat, and to my spirit with something of an air of evil about it. I came around the corner of the house to find that it was lying tauntingly next to its obviously recently killed prey, a small red squirrel - and thinking that the kids would probably be pretty upset at the sight, I figured I should at least throw it in the river behind the house. I cast

away the cat, noticed that the squirrel was still alive, though seemingly paralyzed and with teeth marks across its back, so I picked it up and brought it into the woods. We sat together, the squirrel and I, for probably a couple of minutes before it stirred and scampered off, quite completely whole.

I presume the squirrel was not dead as I had thought. I presume the squirrel was not as injured as I had imagined. But I am certain that that squirrel was staring at certain death with the devil casually admiring its catch. And I am certain that whatever small measure of God's grace allowed me to be there at that moment and claim that squirrel's life was about you. And when the squirrel, quite to my surprise, dashed off into the woods, I was immediately and convincingly overwhelmed with the image of you and the prayers we had offered up, all of us, and of the prayers I continue to have in my heart for you.

That little story reminds me of the certain conviction I had on Saturday. Some might say that if Dick is not healed, that means that Satan won - that our prayers were not answered. I maintain that the only way Satan can "win" is if we lose our faith in God - faith that He is in control and loves us, regardless of the outcome for Dick. That cat thought he had won, but it was a mighty pitiful victory!

****

June 6, 2000

Dick had a difficult night Sunday night; he had lots of abdominal pain, cramping and nausea. He woke up repeatedly, convinced that the medicines were "doing a job" on his stomach. He still felt lousy in the morning, so I went to work a little late - by this time aware that Satan was probably glad to be getting the upper hand after our great day of prayer on Saturday. I had even started to list the prayers that God did not answer: crisis free nights; no more illness; Dick enjoying taking fluids..., but I knew that that was the wrong place to go. By the time I got up in the morning I had made a decision that "I will NOT be Job's wife!" who urged her husband to "curse God and die."

Dick had no pain med all day on Monday, so he was quite miserable by the time of our appointment with Dr. Huberman at 4:00 PM. The doctor switched him to a patch form of pain medicine (Duragesic), which was put on at 5:00. He also gave him some Roxicodone, since it takes time for the patch to begin working, and he prescribed Ativan for nausea.

Although Dick was sleepy all day on Tuesday, he made it to the Underclassman Awards Ceremony tonight. He had to walk very slowly, so even though we left him off as near to the door as possible, we were not there when the ceremony began. Arlene came down looking for us, because Zach's name had already been called. Fortunately, there was an elevator available to get us to the second floor, and Arlene had saved some seats for us. Those directing the ceremony were kind enough to repeat the award for Zach, so we were able to see him receive it - the Dartmouth Book award - as well as several others. By the time the evening was over, Zach had in hand two gold medals (for English and science), a French award (for getting the second highest score in Walpole on the French National Exam) and the Outstanding Junior Award! I know that Dick was glad he made the effort to go out.

Flood:

June 2000 - August 2000

Chapter 22

June 10, 2000

After talking with our families and emailing Ray and Jan, Dick sent this email to friends.

Title: "Going home, just not sure when?"

Greetings to all our prayer partners,

Well, it's been one week since the day of prayer on Saturday, June 3rd. Can't tell you all what a special day that was for us (Nancy, Dick, Jeremy and Zachary), how much we looked forward to it and how much we enjoyed the times together, and to also know that so many other people in so many different places throughout the Boston area and the world were praying for us that day.

As my email of last Monday (June 5th - "Satan is not happy") indicated, things became difficult again (Sunday evening) with the return of pain, nausea and lack of sleep for both me and Nancy. Later on during the week (Wednesday?) things became worse yet in that I started to develop severe double vision. We contacted the neuro-oncologist. He had already moved the previously scheduled June 19th brain scan up to June 9th (Friday morning). He and two other oncologists viewed the images and met with me Friday afternoon to discuss.

The facts are that the three tumors that showed up previously have grown significantly in the past 6 to 8 (?) weeks and that another 5 specs on the older image (previously unnoticed due to their small size) have also grown significantly. That makes at least 8 significantly sized tumors, more or less randomly distributed throughout the brain. Furthermore, there are "many" tiny spots throughout the brain which look like the 5 new tumors did 2 months ago (i.e., tiny, barely perceivable small spots which are too small to categorize at the present time, but it is expected that many of them will grow into significantly sized tumors during the next couple of months.)

The bottom line is that we have pretty much exhausted our treatment options and that we will probably let the disease run its course (i.e., continue to leave my life in God's hands, a good place to be). They expect that I have about 6 months to live, this being the average time span for a person with my condition. They emphasize that there is no way of knowing how the disease will progress, and that the 6 month figure is a guess at how long I have to live. Being an average, I may only have a couple of months to live, or I could live for several more years (if the disease should miraculously go into remission); they just don't know. But there is little left that the doctors have to offer in terms of treatment. They are sorry, but their bag of tricks seems to be empty. Our treatment modality (as of Friday) will move from trying to aggressively fight the disease to treating the symptoms (i.e., pain management - Hospice, etc.) to make me as comfortable as possible in the time that is left.

The most difficult thing for me is thinking about leaving the family behind. I'm not worried about my own going home, but I can't bear the thought of leaving Nancy, Zach, and Jeremy. May I gain the faith to know that God really loves them, even more than I do, and will somehow really make this a blessing in their lives. It is difficult to truly trust God in this area of my life.

Be praying for the family (both our immediate group of four, since we are going through this together, and our extended family: parents, brothers, sisters, and the other close relatives).

And now I get to share two pearls of wisdom that I just received today. One of the many blessings is receiving such things daily from you all and then being able to turn them around and share them with you.
"Cancer is so limited.
It cannot cripple love.
It cannot shatter hope.
It cannot corrode faith.
It cannot eat away peace.
It cannot destroy confidence.
It cannot kill friendship.
It cannot silence courage.
It cannot invade the soul.
It cannot reduce eternal life.
It cannot quench the spirit.
It cannot lessen the power of the Resurrection."
and then this thought as well:
"We never apologize to anyone for depending upon our Creator. We can laugh at those who think spirituality the way of weakness. Paradoxically, it is the way of strength. The verdict of the ages is that faith means courage. All men of faith have courage. They trust their God. We never apologize for God. Instead, we let Him demonstrate, through us, what He can do. We ask Him to remove our fear and direct our attention to what He would have us be. At once, we commence to outgrow fear."

THROUGH THE BARREN TREES

God bless you and may God grant you His peace that passes all understanding:
   Dick and Nancy

****

June 10, 2000

Six months - maybe more, maybe less. Once Dick's double vision started, and with the intermittent nausea, gagging and retching along with the pain, I guess we were not really surprised - and of course we were. What about the clear spinal fluid? The doctor told us that cancer cells don't live long in it; they just pass through it or die so at certain times it could be clear. What about all those prayers and feelings people have that Dick will be healed? I have no answer to that question.

I'm sure it was hard for Dick to tell me what the doctors had said; he wouldn't do it while I was driving. "Just tell me; I know it can't be good," I begged, but he thankfully would not give in to my pleas and waited until we could pull the car over by a pond. Once again, he had gotten the bad news by himself, since Zach had driven him to the doctor's office, and then left. The plan was for me to pick Dick up, but since the doctors decided after Zach left that they would cancel further tests for Dick, he ended up having to just sit and wait for me for about an hour. It wasn't until we pulled the car over by the pond that he could finally speak the words that he dreaded telling me; and oh, how I dreaded hearing them! We cried together there, drove a little further, and then stopped again where we could get out of the car and sit on a bench together, trying to begin to grasp the meaning of what the doctors had told Dick.

It was so hard to tell Zach; we told him while sitting out on our lovely, peaceful deck at suppertime. I'm sure there is never a "good" age to lose one's father, but it is such a critical time in his life now, as he enters his senior year of high school and prepares for college. The tears streamed down Zach's face as he heard words that came as a complete shock to him. He knew his father was sick, but it had never occurred to him that he might die.

Hard as it was to tell Zachary, I think it was even harder to tell Jeremy, since we had to do it over the phone - and his cell phone cut out in the middle of our conversation; apparently it didn't work in his basement apartment, so he had to go out to the parking lot to speak with us. His sobs were heart-wrenching, as he, too, began to understand that

180

the wonders of modern medicine could do no more to "fix" his father. We were grateful that his cousin Liz was with him in Virginia.

How can this be? How can I face being alone when Zach and Dick both leave? I'm not ready for it. I don't think I can ever be ready for it, but I'm getting tired. I hate that Dick has so much pain. I hate that he hasn't been able to feel "normal" for more than two years. I hate that I worry when his breathing is funny at night and I hate that I never get eight hours sleep anymore. But then there is always the grace - to make it through the night without panicking; to wake up - awake; to have people tell us that they love us - so many people!

The words to that Rich Mullins song make so much sense: "Step by step You'll lead me, and I will follow You all of my days..."

****

June 11, 2000
Email from Ray to us

Many thanks for your clear and honest updates, especially the last telling us that you have decided to let the disease run its course. One thing that is clear from all of your communication is how healthy you are - making a difference here between "healthy" and "disease-free". Your spirit (especially), your attitude, your honesty, your approach, your open mourning, your continuing sense of humor all bespeak health. And faith. And The Faith.

I too am glad Eliz is with Jeremy; we cannot be in the States right now, and I'm very thankful Elizabeth can be a closer part of your lives than we can right now. We still, of course, plan to come this summer, arriving Boston Friday 14 July 5:10 PM (oh great, rush hour!) Virgin Atlantic flight #11. Should we still plan to stay with you? Should we involve Mary Ellen and Phil in picking us up? We're still planning the last 2 weeks in July for a trip south, and the last 2 in Aug for a trip west. However, all these plans are tentative.

Please be assured we are praying for you, and know too that we continue to learn from you.

****

181

June 11, 2000
Email from me to Ray and Jan:

Sorry I haven't written much lately. I'm managing to "keep up" but not do some of the extra things I'd like - like notes and journal writing and emails. School ends on Wednesday, so that will help. Meanwhile, a couple of things about your coming here. I'll certainly still plan to pick you up at the airport. We've learned to make plans, realizing that they sometimes need to be changed at the last minute. If we have to make other arrangements at the last minute, we will! Also, yes, you should still plan to stay with us. I'm thinking that other people may want to stop by from time to time this summer, and that will be good, too. Sounds like you'll be away more than you'll be here, but we still look forward to that block of time with you in the beginning of August - or whenever it turns out to be.

Re: transportation: Since we now have 4 cars and 3 drivers, the Caravan is at your disposal. It has a lot of miles on it, but should be able to make a trip south, if you choose to drive. . .

We are planning a brief family vacation for next weekend. Jeremy is expected to fly to Providence on Thursday and then we plan to go to the Cape on Friday to Sunday (the place we went with you guys.) The plan is for Zach to fly back to VA with J on Sunday, and for the 2 of them to visit VA Tech on Monday. Then Zach will bus/train to Baltimore, where I plan to meet him on Tuesday. We plan to see U. Delaware on Wednesday and fly back together. We are arranging for friends to stay with Dick Tuesday night. I'm just not comfortable leaving him alone since unsteadiness and pain levels and nausea and double vision and all are all unpredictable. You could pray that this would all work out for the best. Thanks.

I'm soooooooooo glad that it worked out that you were already planning to come here this summer. It will be good to see your skin, not just your thoughts, and feel your hugs, not just your prayers.

We love you!

Chapter 23

June 12, 2000

Jeremy brought Thor home with him in May. Thor is the little kitten he adopted from an alley behind his fraternity house last fall. The plan is for Thor to stay with us for a year ("365 days only!" Dick says) since Jeremy cannot have cats in his apartment this summer and one of his roommates next year is allergic to cats. Trouble is, the cat is more than a little wild. We tried to keep him as an inside cat, but he has far too much energy to expend inside a house. Also, I attribute his lack of the social graces to the fact that he was abandoned by his mother at a very early age, and then was raised for the first seven months of his life in a fraternity! Seems to me that he has had a decided lack of positive role models in his life - until Dick.

We heard that cats respond well to being squirted with water to prevent them from doing something negative, such as jumping up on tables and destroying plants or sharpening claws on pool tables. I didn't have any little squirt bottles, and apparently Dick couldn't wait, so he went to the basement and brought up our bright yellow three gallon multi-purpose pressurized spray pump. He would sit in his chair in the family room, sprayer at his side, primed to let loose a powerful squirt every time Thor would do something undesirable. Surprisingly, this use was not listed or pictured on the box that the sprayer came in. It was effective, but I decided that for the preservation of the furniture, it might be wise to replace it with something a bit smaller. We now have two small sprayers in different rooms, and the "ultra" version is back in the basement. Dick also has another method of cat training, which he noted in this email to Jeremy:

For about two weeks now I have been using reverse cat psychology on Thor, and I think it is beginning to work. You know how cats act so superior at times, like they will be bothered with you only if they feel like it on their terms.

Well for several weeks now, Thor and I have been home alone most of the time, and all that time I pretty much acted like he wasn't there, even if he started to rub up against my legs.

About five minutes ago while I was typing at the computer, Thor jumped up into my lap and started to purr. So I gave in and touched him, stroking his head and he started to sound more like a motor boat then a cat. We had a few nice moments together before he went crazy again!

****

June 13, 2000
Email from Dick to friends
Title: "Several Specific Prayer Requests"
Greetings in Christ's name,

I have several specific prayer request for the "short term?".

1) Jeremy will be traveling from UVA to home this Thursday evening. Pray for safe traveling and flight from Baltimore to Providence.

2) We (just the four of us) are planning (hoping) to spend about three days at a place on Cape Cod (Father's day weekend). This will be the first time together since the most recent prognosis (i.e., 6 months). We have a lot to catch up on as a family, crying together, praying together, worship. We also hope to have some fun together playing cards, seeing a movie, the beach?

3) Nancy and I are working with both of my oncologists every day trying to find "triggers" and finding the right mixes and doses to control the fatigue, pain, and nausea. Pray that we find the right mix by Friday so that we can make the trip in reasonable comfort.

4) Pray for Jeremy. One of the things we need to discuss / determine is the effect of all this on his summer and fall plans. He has a great job at an architectural firm in VA, and is doing really well at school during the school year, but he also desires to be home with family. I think people need to get on with their lives and not just hang around until I. . . ! We need to make some specific plans. Any decision has to be Jeremy's, but pray that it is something that we all are happy with.

5) Pray for Jeremy's car. Several months a go I bought a used car for Jeremy. He definitely needs it for his job. I thought it to be a pretty good car when I bought it. I had a chance to drive it around for a few weeks myself and have it worked on before he drove it to VA. It's turned out to be a bit of a LEMON. Floods easily and leaves him stranded quite often. He has taken it to mechanics / dealerships, to no avail as of yet. Pray that someone can identify and fix the problem. It's in the shop again right now.

6) Our next big plans are a family reunion (my mother's family) in Syracuse on July 2nd. Pray that we will be up to the 300+ mile trip. There will probably be around forty people attending. Given recent prognosis, this may be the last time I see many of these relatives, at least on this side of glory.

Several times above, I mention the doctor's prognosis which has changed from a small probability of survival, that no one was able to place a specific number on, other than to say there is still a small hope worth fighting for, to an agreement that there wasn't anything more that they could do and it was a reasonable option to let the disease run its course.

Just a note that even though the doctors seem to think my prognosis has changed, Nancy and I do not agree. Several months ago someone asked me what my prognosis was and I responded "Eternal Life". It seems to me that this is still the case.

> *God bless,*
> *Dick*

****

June 16, 2000

We met with Hospice people yesterday morning. Dr. Huberman had suggested that we get involved with them as soon as possible, and we were in full agreement with that plan. After meeting with them, we are even more convinced of the value of this service. They will get equipment (they already got us a wheelchair - the "Breezy 500") and medications; provide social service and pastoral counseling as desired; provide as much nursing service as needed; and provide limited home health aide service if needed for bathing, meal preparation, medication reminders, etc. I think we would need a home health aide only if I return to work in the fall, but in that case we would probably need more than the couple of hours a day that Hospice would provide.

The whole question of whether to return to work or not is a big one. If I do go back and Dick can't be left alone for extended periods (we're near that point now), then we will have to find someone to stay with him. Jeremy says it has crossed his mind to take off a semester or a year. One of his favorite professors lost his father several years ago, when the professor was in his early twenties. The professor counseled Jeremy to consider being at home more so that he does not end up regretting not spending more time with his dad. I am glad that someone he respects - besides his parents - is talking to him about these things and he is really thinking about them. He came home yesterday afternoon. It is good for him to be here. He and Dick have had some long talks about computer stuff - what Jeremy is working on now, and certainly in Dick's field of expertise.

At this point, Jeremy is planning to come home every other weekend during the summer. The Campbell Family Reunion (Dick's family) is planned for July fourth weekend, so Jeremy plans to come up to help us drive out for that.

****

Email from Dick to Anne
Title: "Thursday midnight"

Well, as always, thanks for your prayers. Jeremy arrived safely and we have plans to leave for the Cape today (Friday) before noon. Looking forward to the long weekend together, seafood restaurant at Woods Hole, etc. Now that he lives in Virginia, he's finally ready to try a New England lobster, because his friends in VA can't believe he's never been willing to try one! I'm sure he is open to a new treat.

Thanks for being willing to share your honest opinion. Several people have given us essentially the same counsel, [that perhaps Jeremy should be home for the summer]; however, I think I know Jeremy quite well and he seems very open to the "long weekend together" roughly every two weeks through the summer months. God has already brought Nancy and me through two similar summers these past two years where it's been pretty much Nancy, Dick and God at home for the summer and the boys were both off from home working at camp (counseling and life guarding). If you recall, both of those summers were difficult times for me medically: infections, surgery. I think this summer may be a difficult one physically. I think God knew what He was doing when He removed the kids from home during those months. It took a lot of pressure off of me to not have to worry about constantly putting on the best face to not worry the kids. I think it's the same this summer in that things will be similar and it will help not to continuously be thinking about how my recurring nausea and late night pain is affecting the kids each night.

At this point we are leaving the fall semester completely open; he will decide later on closer to the date when my condition at the time will be better understood.

He and I spent several hours together last night and had a wonderful time.

****

Email from Dick, responding specifically (in capital letters) to an email from his cousin Scott (repeated in italics)

Hello. It's me. Scott. My father forwarded the e-mail you sent to him to us. Wow. It moved me deeply with a mix of emotions. I realize we haven't spoken in a while and to be honest I feel bad. My dad has kept us informed of how you've been doing all along and we have thought and prayed for you guys often.

SOMEHOW WE'VE KNOWN RIGHT ALONG THAT YOU WERE PRAYING FOR US. THANKS!

I guess I've been unsure of how to respond. I wonder if you guys desire privacy or if you would want us to visit. It's difficult to relate or even imagine the depth of your struggles. Anyhow, I'm sorry that I haven't stayed in touch.

I UNDERSTAND THE DIFFICULTY OF KNOWING HOW TO RESPOND. WE ARE STILL STRUGGLING WITH THE DIFFICULTY OF KNOWING HOW TO TELL PEOPLE. LAST SUNDAY I RAN INTO AN OLD FRIEND THAT I HAD NOT SEEN IN A YEAR PLUS IN THE CHURCH PARKING LOT (CHURCH SHOPPING I SUSPECT). HE IS A PROFESSIONAL COUNSELOR, SO I THOUGHT, "HE CAN HANDLE THE TRUTH EASILY ENOUGH", BUT I HAD ALL OF 30 SECONDS TO SAY HELLO AND GOOD-BYE, SO WHEN HE EXTENDED HIS HAND, GLAD TO SEE SOMEONE HE KNEW AND ASKED HOW I WAS DOING (HE ALREADY KNEW THAT I HAVE BEEN IN THIS BATTLE WITH CANCER FOR THE PAST 2 AND ONE HALF YEARS), I JUST RESPONDED "THEY HAVE GIVEN ME 6 MONTHS." HE WAS OBVIOUSLY BLOWN AWAY, AND IT WAS CLEAR, PROFESSIONAL OR NOT, THAT I HAD REALLY, REALLY BLOWN IT. I NEED TO WRITE HIM A CARD THIS WEEK AND ASK FOR HIS FORGIVENESS FOR MY UN-THOUGHTFULNESS IN THE SITUATION.

So now what do I say? I feel like I'm supposed to say something that will touch you. But my God, what can I say? I realize that you are staring death in the face. The reality of folding up your earthly tent and passing thru to the other side must be on your mind continually. Are you still praying for healing or are you just accepting it as the Lord's will?

BOTH. HOPEFULLY, THE TWO ARE THE SAME, BUT WE ARE TRYING TO BE READY FOR ANY OUTCOME, KNOWING WITHOUT DOUBT THAT GOD IS IN CONTROL, BUT CONTINUING TO LET GOD KNOW OUR DESIRE TO BE HEALED.

I really can't imagine saying good-bye to my wife and daughters. Or even worse, them saying bye to me.

THIS IS THE MOST DIFFICULT PART. IT HELPS A LOT THAT THE KIDS ARE REALLY YOUNG ADULTS NOW AND NOT YOUNGER CHILDREN. GOD HAS BLESSED US SO MUCH IN THE PREVIOUS YEARS THAT IT REALLY HELPS TO BE ABLE TO THINK BACK AND REMEMBER. I'M NOT SURE HOW I COULD POSSIBLY HANDLE THE SAME SITUATION EARLY IN MY LIFE, BUT GOD DIDN'T ASK ME TO DO THAT, DID HE?

But at least it's only temporary. I have to admit that a part of me was a little jealous about you going home to be with the Lord. To be enveloped in the bliss of God's eternal love. Safe. Secure. Free from pain. Every trouble and trial swallowed up in His Presence. It's all about Him!

YES, I THINK MY LAST DAY WILL BE A DAY OF GLORY AND HONOR THAT I'M LOOKING FORWARD TO.

I love you guys. May the Lord increase His presence and His love in your home and hearts. I pray that His love would saturate you and overflow. And that many would be impacted by the testimony of your lives.

****

June 17, 2000

What a treat for us all to be here on Cape Cod! We are so fortunate to have generous friends. We are staying in one of Cathy and Chuck's lovely little cottages. They had invited us to stay here - as well as in two other of their cottages - in the past, but this time I was the one who brought up the idea of using one of the cottages for this special little family vacation, and Cathy quickly agreed to my request.

The cottage, named "Seaglass", is the third to last house on a street that ends at the bay, so the view is lovely. Despite its diminutive size, the cottage itself has everything one could need: a bedroom with a double bed; another with bunk beds; an open area which includes a living room / kitchen / dining area; a loft with several more mattresses; a wrap around porch (which we found to be the preferred place for eating); and my favorite thing: an outdoor shower Unquestionably the best part of the shower is the absence of a ceiling or roof, so that one can look up at the trees and sky while one showers. On a hot day, one avoids that whole steamed-up-bathroom situation. Lovely.

The weather this weekend was not expected to be great - especially today. We were expecting a thunderstorm this afternoon and not especially outstanding weather generally. Well, either that prediction was wrong or God changed His mind, because although it is a bit overcast now (7:00 PM), the weather has been <u>beautiful</u> yesterday and today.

****

June 18, 2000

I hate it when Dick and I argue - especially now. He got up in the middle of the night last night and was scratching / picking at himself. He seemed really restless, and did not want to empty his ostomy bag. I thought (in my sleepy state) that he (in his sleepy state) was trying to remove the bag instead of just "burping" it to let the gas out. I told him to go to the bathroom to do what he needed to do, and then I was concerned if he was really alert and able to stay up on his own. While he was up, he took pain medication, but he didn't really seem to be in pain.

Anyway, the upshot of all of this is that it is very hard - especially at night - to know how much I should be helping and correcting Dick and how much I should just leave him alone. His double vision and unsteadiness concern me, but he (understandably) resents it if I "take over" too much. I want to be with him all the time - or at least be sure that someone is with him - but it is tiring to always be concerned and especially to never get a full night's sleep.

We had a short unproductive talk then, and then later we had a longer more productive one. I had wanted to go up to New England Frontier Camp for one weekend to help the nurse there, and I figured that Jeremy could stay with his dad when I went, but Dick does not want me to go away while Jeremy is here. He wants family time - however many of us can be together as possible. He also misunderstood me, thinking I wanted to go away for several weekends and said, "If I die soon, you'll feel terrible that you were up at camp instead of spending those weekends with me." True enough. He also offered a good suggestion for me to get some more sleep; he suggested that maybe some night when Jeremy is home, Jeremy could "take the night shift", sleeping in the room with Dick so that I could go elsewhere in the house and get a full night's sleep. Good idea.

After we worked out those things, we spent a while crying; it is <u>so</u> hard to think of his leaving. I know it is not his choice, but he feels badly (guilty?) that he is abandoning us - but he's <u>not</u>. It's just that God has a different idea for his location. Still, it is so hard... I don't want him to go. Yet, by God's grace I am able to have the privilege of walking the path to death with Dick - with joy along the way.

****

June 19, 2000
Email from Dick to friends
Title: "Great Father's Day Weekend!"

Thanks to all who were praying for us this past weekend. This is just a quick note to let you know that we had a great weekend. Jeremy arrived Thursday evening as planned, and we were off to Cape Cod at noon on Friday as planned. The one and one half hour trip to the Cape went fairly well, even though I was quite tired upon arrival.

I took several short naps while at the Cape, felt nauseated at various times, but these times always passed relatively quickly and without the need for medical intervention (didn't even need to make a single phone call, special since we had called at least once per day before leaving).

I had a wonderful lobster dinner (Father's day celebration, Saturday night, restaurant right on the pier at Woods Hole, watching the ferries arriving from the various Islands), Jeremy enjoyed his flay melon [filet mignon]; Zach and Nancy's dinners were seafood dinners, not all that great, but no major complaints.

Saturday was beautiful weather (even though the prediction was for heavy rains in the afternoon) and we spent several hours at the ocean beach in Falmouth, then had lunch, took a nap, went to the 3:30 showing of MI: 2, nap, and then a late dinner (I enjoyed a great kettle of lobster stew).

Sunday we woke up, packed, went to breakfast, and drove the boys to Providence, RI for a flight to Baltimore. They then made the 3 hour car trip safely to Charlottesville VA and we (Nancy and I) drove back to an empty nest (except for our dog, Casper, and Jeremy's cat, Thor)!

Note: plans have been made for Jeremy to come home and spend long weekends here in Walpole, approximately every other week through the summer months. Everyone seems comfortable with this decision. No plans have been made for next semester, for either Jeremy or Nancy. We will wait until much later in the summer to see how things are going and make plans at that time depending on my condition then. Please keep this in prayer for the family, and especially for Jeremy and Nancy as they decide what to do about work and school.

Thanks again for your prayers; everything went really well and wanted you all to know right away.

Chapter 24

June 22, 2000
Email to us from Kathy

First off, thanks for keeping us informed all along about what's happening with your family. Some e-mails are pretty hard to read, most all are inspiring and uplifting, some make us laugh . . . but all help us to still feel a part of your lives. And your letters make us feel better, or at least not quite so helpless, because we know that at least we can add our prayer support to the many prayers you are already receiving, and that together all those prayers are helping to get you through these challenging times.

I told Tim this past week that in one sense I am a little envious of your family, because your circumstances have pushed you to make the most of your times together, and have helped you all express to each other your love and concerns and deepest feelings. Many families (ours included) can go for long periods of time without deep and meaningful encounters. And so, although I don't envy you your circumstances, I know that God has used Dick's illness and prognosis to bring you all closer than ever together and closer than ever to God. Pretty amazing what blessings can come from such an ugly thing as cancer.

I don't think it's denial that makes me convinced that it's not "all over" yet. I think God loves to bless and surprise us, so I'm still holding on to that hope for you guys. But then, as Dick says, Eternal Life is not such a bad prognosis either! I know whatever happens after death is more wonderful than anything we've yet been able to imagine with our small brains. Did you by chance see the recent TV special on the life of Dietrich Boenhoffer? In the last scene, as he's heading toward the gallows, the Nazi officer who has been harassing him all along says "So, this is the end." And the last line of the program is Dietrich Boenhoffer saying, simply, "No, it's not..."

I hope the July 2 reunion is just as good for you as your Father's Day weekend on the Cape. As always, know that our prayers are with you all.

****

Dick responded to that email:

Nancy and I have been talking a lot the past several weeks, and realize that a lot of people would think that a 6 month "sentence" would be a very difficult thing to live with. However, we are finding it a very special blessing. Instead of just passing away quickly in one's sleep or in an auto accident, or dying from some disease such as Alzheimer's disease that puts years of great stress on the family (as we well know from my father's recent death after 8 years with the disease), we have been given this 6 month grace period (more of less?) in order to say good-bye to our loved ones (friends and family). People are coming over to the house for a time of prayer, a time to grieve together, a time to remember together, a time to laugh together, a time to say good-bye (for now, until we see each other again!). We also have time together for these special family mini trips / vacations / reunions, etc. Each day contains its physical pain, but so far the doctors and hospice continue to be a great help.

Your insight into the situation is right on target.

****

June 23, 2000

We've continued to make adjustments as Dick's condition is changing, and the modifications have really helped the days to go more smoothly. Before we went to the Cape, the boys moved Dick's computer and computer desk to the living room so that he does not have to keep climbing up and down the stairs to get to it. We also started sleeping on the futon in the family room, both to keep Dick's life "stair-free" and because the new super firm mattress we got to ease his lower back pain has proved to be too firm for his shoulder.

I flew to Baltimore as planned to meet Zachary for a visit to the University of Delaware. That went well, though Zach didn't get the impression that "this is definitely the place for me." The best part of that trip was that Dick fared well without us. Bobbie and Carolyn both came to stay with him while I was gone (Bobbie being the nurse, and Carolyn the cook). When I called him from Delaware to see how things were going, he said, "Great! Just like living in community again." I hadn't been worried about him, but was pleased to hear that he had actually enjoyed himself.

I was gone only one night, and the following night we both attended a business meeting at church, where Dick presented a project on which he has been working: the design of a web page for our church. He had taken a survey of people in the church, asking about their use of the internet and their interest in using a church web page or helping with its creation and maintenance. He has really done quite a bit of work on this project, and he gave a very clear presentation. Most people were quite enthusiastic about it, but there does not currently seem to be someone to take over the project when Dick is no longer able to do it.

Last night our neighbor Debbie came to visit while we were sitting on the deck after supper. She wanted to tell us that she had recently learned that her mother is dying, and she also wanted to bring over some holy water that a friend of hers had brought back from Lourdes. She asked if she could share it with Dick - not necessarily for healing, but for peace. She offered it to me, but I suggested that she "do" it. I wouldn't have known what to do, but she kindly touched his forehead with it. What a thoughtful thing to share with us, especially in the midst of her own pain.

This morning we saw Dr. Huberman. Unfortunately, Dick had severe pain just before we got to the office building and for nearly an hour until his pain medication helped, but other than that, he felt reasonably well today. I had a number of things that I needed to discuss with Dr. Huberman, including asking him to fill out disability forms, but rather than being annoyed with me, he actually said he thought that Dick was lucky to have me! Nice man.

After the appointment, since Dick was feeling well, we stopped at the Arboretum for a stroll with Dick in his wheelchair. We had passed the Arnold Arboretum - a wonderful tree park - dozens and dozens of times on all our trips to and from the hospital, but there never seemed to be the right time to stop. We actually did stop the day we got "the news" about Dick's latest prognosis, but at that point Dick didn't have the wheelchair, so he did not have the energy to go very far. Today we had a very pleasant walk - and a good workout for me, since there are some hilly paths in the Arboretum. After that, we stopped at a favorite restaurant - Bertucci's - where Dick feasted on sausage soup. It was a great day, but he was tired when we reached home, so he lay down for a nap. I decided to use the time when he was sleeping to go out to get a few things for him.

When I arrived home a half an hour or so later, I was completely amazed to see him driving away from the house in our minivan! He hasn't driven a car in weeks, and his double vision is quite severe now. I jumped out of my car to yell and flag him down to stop, and thankfully he noticed me and stopped. He got out of the van - wearing slippers instead of shoes, and no eye patch (the eye patch has been helping the double vision.) It was obvious that he had left in a hurry, because he had not shut or locked the door to the house.

When I reached him, he said, "Okay, you can drive. Just get in. We have to go."

"Where?" I asked.

"Some guy called," he answered. "He was very insistent. I have to meet him at Jimmy's [Pizzeria - about a mile down the road]. He's got a package for me. Just trust me. He sounds like he's on a mission for someone - it's not from him. I think it's probably just a get well card from someone, but I told him I'd meet him."

I was ready to go to the end of the street and around the block and back home again - convinced that Dick had either had a very vivid dream, or else the tumor was pressing on the cognitive portion of his brain and he was "losing it", or else there was some crazy guy at Jimmy's!

I suggested that I wasn't going to go to Jimmy's, but Dick was insistent. He reassured me, "Don't worry; he's not going to have a gun or anything, but he really wanted me to come. Just drive in Jimmy's parking lot, and if he's not there, we'll just go back home."

So we did. We pulled in the parking lot.

"There!" Dick exclaimed. "The red truck. He said he'd be in a red truck."

I didn't see it at first, but there was a red van, with a man obviously watching for us. We pulled up next to him and Dick identified himself as Richard Kline. (I would have preferred that this guy not know our names, but it was too late to think of that!) I got out, and the fellow started to hand me a package, but made it clear that I would have to sign for it .

"Are you his daughter?" he asked. (I decided this guy was okay after all!) It became quickly obvious that the package was no get well card, but the pain medication for which Dr. Huberman had faxed orders to Hospice, who had then forwarded them to a special pharmacy that delivers.

On the way home, I was finally able to piece together the story. This fellow in the red van was the pharmacy delivery person, and apparently did not know where our home was, and perhaps did not have a map or know how to follow one. (It appeared that English was not his primary language.) He had phoned Dick to get directions, waking him from a sound sleep. He asked Dick, "Where are you?" and Dick reportedly replied, "I'm at the other end of a wireless phone. Where are you?" The delivery person apparently kept saying something that sounded to Dick like "red man", though in hindsight, it was probably "red van." In Dick's sleepy state, he apparently decided that it would be easier just to meet the fellow at Jimmy's - a decision that he perhaps might <u>not</u> have made had he been more awake!

****

June 28, 2000
Email from Nancy to friends
Title: "Nancy's News"

I am so very aware that when you think of and pray for Dick, I am included in those thoughts and prayers, so I wanted to thank you all again, and let you know how I am doing.

I agree with Dick that the Cape weekend was great. Two things he didn't mention: We all gave him clothes for Father's Day, but the most exquisite article was the Perfect Hat that Zach had bought for him on Newbury Street (for you non-Bostonians, we are talking ELITE here.) Great choice. The other thing Dick didn't mention was the spending of the Family Laundered Money. For years we have been collecting the money that ends up in the washer and dryer (along with a few stray coins from couch cushions, etc.) to be used for some great family treat (Ed. RK - please don't leak the information about the laundered money to the IRS!). We brought it to the Cape and the perfect EXTRAVAGANT expense opportunity presented itself: an extra large (refillable) popcorn at the movie theater! Add the $1 we spent for parking at the beach to the $6.99 for the popcorn and it was pretty darn close to the $8.29 we had saved. (Thankfully, it was a matinee, or I think there might have been people behind me in the popcorn line who might not have appreciated my counting out nickels and pennies to pay!)

Such are the little things that make up life and deserve to be enjoyed. Thus, Dick and I have decided in the midst of our uncertain future, that we must live life fully in the present, and remember to trust God for the future. We've certainly cried plenty, and there will no doubt be many more tears to come, but to waste time worrying about tomorrow means that we'll miss what we have today. So, we get out the Breezy 500 wheelchair (affectionately known as "Breezy" or "the Breeze") and we take our 1/2 hour walk with the dog each day and enjoy the sunshine and each other. Dick's sleep schedule is a bit odd, so we have many a great late night chat. I'm delighted to be off work for the summer, and we continue to enjoy times with friends. There is much that Dick has to teach me about finances and the computer and countless other things around the house that have traditionally been his territory, so our days are full. Hospice is a great support, and with the modifications that have been made (medications for pain and nausea; moving things so Dick no longer has to go upstairs; using the wheelchair for energy conservation), the past several days have gone quite smoothly.

We hope and pray for a good trip to Syracuse this weekend for his family reunion. We're glad Jeremy will be driving out with us for that.

I continue to be amazed at God's grace that we are able to walk this difficult path with a good measure of joy. Thank you again for your thoughts and prayers.

****

June 30, 2000

Most of the time Dick seems completely alert and oriented, but sometimes he makes comments that are not reality based. One morning he woke up and said, "The Pope is dead." I don't remember the whole conversation, but he also said something about space balls. He feels that the world is made up of thousands of space balls and that he somehow generates them. He made a comment something to the effect that, "If you wake up in the morning and notice a bunch of broken space balls on the bed, you'll know the Pope is dead." A few days later he said that the space balls are still around sometimes. "I have to nurture the space balls. Sometimes when I get up at night and go to the bathroom, it's like another space ball has died." When Dick makes comments like these, he seems completely aware that these are things that are known to him and not to me. It is actually not particularly upsetting to either of us, but I am glad that he feels free to talk to me about things like space balls.

Zachary left three days ago to counsel and lifeguard at New England Frontier Camp again. He has his own car, so he will be able to come home more often than he might have without easy transportation. I'm going to miss him, but I'm glad he is going.

****

Dick continues to refer people to the Kline Family web page, but he just updated it with the following explanation:

The last sentence of this web page used to be: "The story is not over yet, but that's all there is for now. I will add further information to this archive in the future as the story progresses." However, it is beginning to look like the story is nearly over, at least if any story is really ever over. So I probably will not be making further large additions to this web site. Another reason is because my health is failing and even this last update took a tremendous amount of energy for me. I was hoping that working on the computer would be one last enjoyment (hobby) that I would be able to enjoy to nearly the end, but it has become clear that even that requires too much energy to do anything very extensive. Therefore I have to switch to a very low maintenance mode as far as the web site is concerned. In the future, I will rely on the prayer list emails (both sent and replies to) as the main source of information on our condition, developments, needs, and requests. I'll also use the space beneath this horizontal line to archive the emails in chronological order so that people in the future can see "the rest of the story."

****

July 2, 2000

"Everything's falling apart - but that's to be expected at the end of time." That was Dick's comment as he awakened from a sound sleep after a big day, and he felt that he couldn't "put it all together" or "connect reality." He <u>seemed</u> clear - cognizant of what we had done today and of our current plans - but said "two and two don't make three yet, but that's okay. . ."

Today was the Campbell Family Reunion - Dick's mother's family. The reunion went really well, though the weekend started off a bit "shaky". The only flight I could get for Jeremy to come home this weekend left Baltimore at 9:30 yesterday morning - Saturday; there were no Friday night flights available at all. That meant he had to get up at 5:00 AM in order to get to the airport on time, and even though he arrived approximately forty minutes before flight time, they "bumped" him - said that there was no room on the flight for him! He called us promptly to discuss the situation, since we had planned to leave for Syracuse shortly after picking him up in Providence at 10:35 AM. The next flight out of Baltimore was not until 1:20 PM, and there was no guarantee that he would get on that. We told him that it was okay for him to go back to

Virginia instead of waiting for the next flight, but he made the decision to wait. As it turned out, he did get on that next flight, and also got a voucher for $266 for future air travel, since the airline had withdrawn his reservation. He arrived home a little tired, but ready and willing to set out right away for the reunion.

We had a nice ride out to Syracuse, with lots of time to talk. Jeremy told us that he is currently thinking that he will most likely come home this fall instead of going back to school, even though he would not be able to make up his classes the next summer and would end up being a year behind his classmates. The professor that had spoken to him before told Jeremy essentially that he did not want to see him back at school in the fall, again encouraging him to spend time with his father while he can. Jeremy is willing to come home and work construction or maybe get a job as a waiter in the evenings so that he could care for Dick during the day if I decide to go back to work.

One thing Jeremy and Dick talked about during the car trip to Syracuse was a new (top secret!) project to work on together to make them millionaires. It is some kind of an invention that actually sounds quite plausible to them both. Wouldn't that be a hoot? Dick stops working because of cancer, but then is cured by a miracle and becomes a millionaire from an invention that he develops in his "free time" while out of work!

Today was a good day, with lots of relatives eager to see Dick. He did not want to be the center of attention, so we arrived a little bit late to the reunion. (I offered to go pantless to take the focus off of him, but we decided to forgo that plan!) The day was beautiful, the food was delicious (Dick especially liked the locally made hot dogs), and there were many good conversations, but leaving was tough. Dick got tired, and as he sat in the car waiting to leave, the family all came to him to say good-bye. There were lots of tears, and seeing people cry often makes other people cry, so it was rather heartbreaking. It was a good-bye unlike any the family had experienced before, knowing that most of them would not see Dick again this side of Heaven. Grandma, John, his wife Susan, and their daughter Elizabeth do plan to come out to visit later in the summer. That will be good.

****

199

July 3, 2000

Last night Dick awoke in the middle of the night and talked for about forty-five minutes about what was on his mind. "My view of reality - somehow my view of reality did not include existence beyond July 3. I'm clear as a bell, but I can't explain why I felt or believed that way. When I woke up, I felt like I was in a life boat, and the world was two dimensional with a thin third dimension. I wouldn't have put a date on it before, but for the past couple of weeks I've been having trouble explaining reality or my view of reality was changing. I felt that life was predetermined - like I just was pushing buttons - that I really had no decisions to make, like about what I'd have for breakfast; I'd just push a button and I'd have eggs."

He went on talking like this, indicating that somehow things were more clear to him than they had been, but it certainly did not sound clear to me!

We arrived back from Syracuse with more wonderful emails awaiting us on the computer. This one came from Beth. Title: "I'm just thinking of you"

I've just reread through your web-site. I want to be available without being intrusive. I wish for you to have the peace that passes understanding. I don't understand why this is happening. In reading your web-site, it is obvious that you have the support of many and so are blessed. How sad that so many others face such travail without the tangible support of others. Somehow, however, I think that everyone has an Intercessor. And in the midst of this earthly crowd, Dick, you are not alone, even when the email, postal service and phone is silent, and the house is quiet, you are not alone. The fact is that not one of us fellow travelers can take away your suffering. But, you are not alone. He is with you. He loves you more than any mortal can (hard to believe that there is someone greater than Nancy, Jeremy, or Zachary, isn't it?) I marvel at how you and Nancy can now enjoy life while home alone and when you have time with your two marvelous sons. And how you can see "the beauty of the sky through the bare 'wintry' branches" of this time of your lives. Nancy, you are an example of the greatest gift for your family: caring for Dick in all his miseries, planning for get-aways with your family, making your home a place of refuge for those who are in need. I love you both. I am privileged to know you. You are a living example of "A Grief Observed"; thank you for sharing your life with me and so many others. I weep with you and I will never stop to pray for the

miracle of the restoration of health for you. I cling to this life, but I believe there is a greater Life ahead for all of us.
Beth

****

July 4, 2000
Jeremy left this morning. It sure was nice to have him along for the trip.
Before we went away, Barb and Bob had contacted us about hosting a July fourth barbecue here for however many of our friends or family we chose to invite. They brought <u>everything</u> for the gathering, including food, serving dishes, aprons and instruments for grilling - even recycling and trash barrels! We had invited an interesting mix of people: some from the house church we were part of many years ago, and several others that we have known from various times in our lives. One fellow who was invited but couldn't come brought over bags full of fireworks to add a festive touch to the celebration.

****

July 6, 2000
It really bothers me when Dick has disordered thinking. Most of the time he is very clear with only minor short term memory lapses ("Did I already take my pills?") but he just had another one of those episodes like the space balls incident or the "reality" monologue. Once again, it occurred after a deep sleep. He had just slept a couple of hours and was apparently hungry when he awoke, so he decided to fix himself a snack. I was downstairs in the basement, and when I came up, the microwave oven was on. He said he was going to have a hot dog (left over from lunch) and then go back to bed. I asked if he wanted a roll, but he declined, and seeming a little annoyed that I had asked, he took some bread out of the refrigerator. I asked again if he wanted bread instead of a roll with his hot dog, and he again appeared a bit irritated with me. He fished around in the bread bag for a moment, then closed the bag without getting any bread. About this time, the microwave shut off and he went to get his hot dog, but there was nothing in the microwave oven. I found the hot dog on a plate in the refrigerator, and we heated it up. He declined a roll, instead eating it with a fork, along with some grapefruit juice. He then started a discourse on why it was so important that he eat

201

this hot dog. He said it was important to him and important to me (?!) - that I had "made that very clear" - and then he went on to talk about the existence of the hot dog. I didn't say much, except to point out that I didn't really care if he ate the hot dog, but I would like for him to take his pills. He did not object.

This little exchange did not last very long - probably less than fifteen minutes - but after Dick went back to bed, I was left in tears. Even though he is completely "with it" most of the time, this was the second incident of this kind in less than a week. Frankly, it scares me a little and saddens me a great deal. It makes me feel as though I am losing him piece by piece. Some of the pieces are more difficult to lose than others. Losing his being the major wage earner was okay, because he still gets disability payments and I have an income and we have adequate savings. Losing him as the designated driver was not a problem - I'm a lousy back seat driver anyway; I like being in control of the car. Losing him as handyman and dishwasher was not so bad - Zach and I can pick up the slack.

The first really difficult loss was the touch one. We certainly still touch, and we still sleep in the same bed, but it used to be that the best part of sleeping in the same bed was snuggling together to fall asleep. That became more difficult as Dick became more uncomfortable, so I had gotten used to just touching our feet together, when one night he came over to my side of the bed and started to caress me. It immediately made me cry to realize how rare that was - how long it had been - and how it probably would never be a big part of our marriage again. Tough loss #1.

Tough loss #2. Right now we communicate about everything: present, future, past; concerns, plans, sorrows. Sometimes the things we talk about aren't easy, but we TALK. When his mind goes to these other places - like with the reality thing and the hot dog - I'm left out. No one has seen this except me, since these times usually occur after a deep sleep. This makes me feel incredibly ALONE!! I have dear friends who have said, "Call me anytime - day or night." That is so sweet, but what would I say? I just want to cry until my husband comes back!

One day I asked Sandy, the hospice nurse, how she thought Dick might die. I expected her to say something about his liver or lungs, describing how his body would shut down, but instead she said that often people get to the point where they are just ready to go; they have accomplished what they want, and they don't want to go on living the way they have become, so they die! On the other hand, she said that some people get to the point where they are ready to go, but they "hang on" in a coma for weeks.

Dick does have a number of things he wants to do: start a web page for church; make sure our finances are in order; complete notebooks of memories of his life for each of the boys and me. He still spends a lot of time on the computer, and even though it is becoming more difficult for him to do computer related tasks, we are both grateful for the structure that his list of projects brings to his days.

Chapter 25

July 6, 2000
Email to Ray and Jan regarding their impending visit:
    Figured I'd better write once more before you leave so you know that I DID get your email and DO plan to meet you at Logan on Fri. 7/14 at 5:10 at Virgin Atlantic gate or baggage or whatever. J is due in 1/2 hr after you in Providence, but a friend of his will pick him up. We'll let you dog tired people just go to bed if you want. Zach plans to come in the next day also - doesn't want to miss the action!
    I had this one funky thought. For you, Jan. Remember - or did I mention - the possibility of the nuclear Downing Family (i.e. Harry, Ebba, Mary Ellen, Ray and Nance) going to Camp of the Woods in early August for 1-2 nights? I'm not willing to leave Dick alone over night, and maybe this is a dumb idea anyway, but if it worked, how would you feel about staying here with Dick? He's open to it, but I just mention it as something to think about. Mary Ellen hasn't made reservations yet, and we don't even know what is available, so it's just possibly a possibility.
    Well, we're certainly looking forward to seeing you all!!!

****

July 13, 2000
    Monday, Tuesday and Wednesday this week there was a School Nurse Conference in Boston. It seemed as though it would be a good thing for me to attend along with several of the other Walpole school nurses, but I was not willing to leave Dick alone for the whole time that I was gone. We decided to take two cars into Boston each day in case I had to leave early, and I arranged for different people to visit Dick each morning and afternoon. Many people have expressed a desire to spend some time with him, so this seemed to be a good way to arrange that. I posted my cell phone number by each of our home phones, and I kept my fully charged cell phone with me at all times.
    On Monday morning I also informed Dick (after much agonizing thought about how to handle this) that I would be making the car keys inaccessible to him. Although I knew he would not drive if he were thinking clearly, I was concerned that he might try to drive if he were disoriented or "cloudy" (NB. the big red van incident.) I put his keys and

the spare set of car keys upstairs in the bottom of my underwear drawer. Dick had not been upstairs in several days, so I assumed that the bedroom was a safe place to relocate the keys. I had asked Carolyn's son Corey to call Dick at 9:00 to see if he might like to go out to breakfast, since that is one of Dick's favorite things to do. Since our friends John and Janet were to visit at 12:00, Dick's day would be quite full, and there would really be no need for him to drive anywhere at all.

Well, there I was, in the far front of a big sloping auditorium type classroom - rear exit only - in the middle of a lecture - when the lovely strains of "Ode to Joy" broke forth from the recesses of my purse. My phone was ringing. I scooted out of the room as quickly as possible, but not quickly enough to answer it before the ringing stopped. Since Dick and the boys are the only ones who know the cell phone number, I assumed that the call was either from Dick or it was a wrong number (that had happened once before in another auditorium.) I called Dick to find that, yes, he had called me, because he was looking for the car keys! He said that Corey was going to take him out, and he wanted Corey to drive the van. We did not discuss then or later why they couldn't use Corey's car; I expect he would have said it was because he thought it would be easier to get the wheelchair in and out of the van. Anyway, I explained where the keys were, emphasizing that Corey, not Dick, should retrieve the keys, since stair climbing often precipitated vomiting for Dick. I was a bit embarrassed at the thought of this twenty-something young man rifling through my underwear drawer, but what could I do? Dick agreed to let Corey get the keys, but when I called later, Dick informed me that Corey had come late, so Dick went up and got the keys himself. I'm so glad that he didn't either vomit or fall!

On Tuesday, I opted to go late to the conference, since Dick had had a period of disorientation during the night, and I was uncomfortable leaving him alone in the morning. Also, the visitor we had planned for the morning had not seen him in some time, and I did not think it was fair to leave her alone with him if there might be any problems. The person who was to come in the afternoon had canceled, so once again I called Carolyn, and sweetheart that she is, she agreed to come for a couple of hours in the afternoon so that I could go in for part of the conference.

Wednesday went well. Dick was feeling better than he had been, and was a bit less "foggy" and tired, since we had cut back on the Duragesic Patch pain medication. His visitors, Paul and Bob, came as planned, and Sandy, the hospice nurse, arrived just before I returned home. She already had called Dr. Huberman regarding further medication changes. Dr. Huberman is going to increase the Decadron and have Dick try morphine tablets instead of Roxicodone.

****

July 21, 2000

Ray and Jan arrived from Africa as planned a week ago. Jeremy also came on Friday, and Zach was here from Saturday to Sunday. Tim brought Zach a <u>most</u> unique (and very much appreciated) gift from Kenya: a varnished elephant turd! Ray recounted his concern that along with the questions that are usually asked at Customs, "Are you carrying anything for anyone? Have you left your luggage unattended at any time?" they might ask, "Are you carrying any elephant turds?"

Ray, Jan and Tim left Monday afternoon in our Caravan for points south - to see Liz and then go to Tennessee. They expect to be back at the beginning of August.

Tuesday night Dick's mom, his brother John and his niece Kristen arrived. What a great visit! They stayed until Thursday, and John spent most of the day Wednesday, with Kristen's help, building a wheelchair ramp to the front door. He also built a little step to make it easier for Dick to go out to the deck. What a difference these things make! Other accommodations that have helped are a shower chair and a commode that Sandy arranged to have delivered so that showers can be more relaxing for Dick and the commode can serve as an elevated seat for the toilet.

I was <u>so</u> glad that Kristen and Dick's mom came to visit, although I know it was not easy for either of them. I can't imagine being in his mother's shoes: living 300 miles away from her son when he is dying. I wonder if I were in her situation if I would want to go to my son and hover over him - trying to soak up every second I could have with him - and assume that because I was his mother I could best meet his needs, but she was not like that at all. She was extremely supportive and encouraging of me - repeatedly telling me how grateful she is that her son is married to me. What a special gift that was to me! She also expressed her willingness to help in any way possible; buying great "take out" meals was a nice part of that.

****

206

July 22, 2000

This morning Dick and I worked to install a new printer for the computer. The one that we had bought with the new computer just a few months ago died. We really didn't want to take the time to send it back and wait for it to be fixed under warranty, because we want a printer that works now, while Dick is still able to use it. Computer work is difficult for me because it is an area in which I am not very skilled; that has always been Dick's department. However, I offered to help because I really want for the computer to work well for Dick; he deserves that little bit of enjoyment. He had tried to install the printer himself, but due to his self-reported "fogginess", he had not been successful. I had also tried to help once, but I, too, failed. Today we followed the step by step instructions: I read and Dick did. That went well, but because of the two earlier incomplete installation attempts, the computer thinks we have three printers, and it keeps saying "fatal error" (I hate that message!) It did manage to print one document with printer three, and then printed another five page document three times. The situation clearly needs more work.

This afternoon, after a long morning nap, Dick declared that the day was for me to do whatever I wanted. We did some banking and then went to the mall, where he bought me a diamond earring. I had been hinting for one for a long time, but he hadn't gotten the hint. I finally stated that I was going to get a fourth hole made - in the top of my right ear - for a diamond. He agreed to come with me and buy the earring. My plan is for it to always be there: it is from the man I love, and "diamonds are forever".

So, most of the day was good, but then I made the mistake of trying to plan the end part. I thought that after Dick took a nap we could take a walk and then have supper and watch a movie; but he had a lot of trouble waking up, had shoulder pain, and didn't want supper. I have to face that he may wake up in the middle of the night, and that will be his day.

I can rationally recognize that life is different, but it is still sometimes difficult to accept that: my life is not my own; control is an illusion; planning is somewhat futile; and day and night are irrelevant to one with cancer on mind-altering medications. I had better learn to be FLEXIBLE!

****

207

July 23, 2000
Email from Dick to Jim in response to Jim's request, "Let me know how things are going."
Very busy. Trying to get everything done in time. It's amazing how much there is to do. Also having a great time with family, reunions, friends, get-togethers, etc. Printer on computer broken which is a major pain in the butt. Jeremy coming home next weekend for the weekend and will probably help me in this as well as many other small areas. Concentration and pain is a problem, but still mostly under control (morphine) at the moment. Very pleased with level of care provided by Hospice.

****

July 24, 2000
Dick sent an email to Jeremy, Zachary and me telling us that he felt that we should not worry about finances. He has made good provision for us and he reminded us that "of course, our God owns the cattle on a thousand hills." How sweet of him to be thinking of us in such a concrete and practical way! Besides that, we have signed papers so that I have Power of Attorney for Dick, just in case that is needed. We are also in the process of talking with a lawyer friend, our financial advisor and my brother-in-law Phil (a banker, so he has good input) about making sure our finances are in order. This is really not my area of interest or expertise, so it is rather anxiety producing, but Dick (I am sure wisely) feels it is important for his family's future that this be addressed now.

****

July 27, 2000
Email from me to friends
Title: "Update"
It has been a long time since I have sat down in front of the computer - both because we have been so busy this summer and also because Dick spends so much of his time here that it is hard to get a word in edgewise, so to speak!
Mostly we are doing well. We have seen a LOT of friends and family over the past several weeks. Clearly, Dick is such a special person that people want to spend time with him while they can. This has served to be a good thing for us, as we have little time to sit around and

wallow in sadness. Obviously the sadness is there, but God has been so good in allowing us to enjoy things each day.

Most days we walk (well, Casper and I walk, and Dick rides in Breezy 500, which serves to keep us all at the correct temperature as long as I dress very lightly and Dick dresses warmly!) We have thoroughly enjoyed the exceptional number of sunny but not-too-hot days this summer. Besides the walks and visits and appointments, Dick has been very busy with getting his affairs in order - financial; thinking about house repairs; writing some memories for the boys and me; and planning his funeral.

We continue to make modifications so that he can get the most out of the strength that he has left. His brother built a wonderful wheelchair ramp out the front door - just in time, as he could no longer walk up the stairs. Saturday we expect to have another friend install bars in the bathroom for easier movement and support. We continually are assessing and modifying pain medication to achieve the right balance between pain control and clarity of thought, since both are equally important. This is going pretty well.

Having a terminal illness unfortunately does not exempt one from the normal irritations of life, such as broken computer printers, but we hope to soon have the new printer in good working order. (We're hoping that this weekend Jeremy will be able to help Dick get rid of that frightening blue "fatal error!" screen that comes up every time we try to print!)

Jeremy continues to come home every other weekend, and will most likely take a year off of school, initially to be here with Dick, and then return to VA to continue (hopefully) to work at the architecture / building firm where he is this summer.

Zach will be away at camp till mid August (that has been very good for him) though he plans to come home for a few days next week. He has made the decision to not play soccer this fall so he can be at home more. We are very grateful for the maturity and care that both boys have shown.

The really good news Dick got last week was that the project he began work on 5 years ago (his "baby") is actually working! He went in to work last week and saw a demonstration of a computer chip for which he was the chief architect. It is used in telephone communications somehow - apparently has lots of potential applications - and other than that it is completely beyond my comprehension. It is about 1 1/4" square (including its 420 teensy connectors) and contains 33 MILLION *transistors. Doesn't make sense to me. (For some reason it makes me think of that question, "How many angels can fit on the head of a pin?") Anyway, what a very special gift for him to be able to see this project come to fruition while he is still alive.*

Well, I just wanted to give you an update. As you can see, things have changed, and yet they haven't. We are aware that, barring a miracle, our time together on this earth is much more limited than we would have liked, but we continue to experience God's daily Amazing Grace, and we are resting in His unfailing love.

Love to you, with thanks for your continued thoughts and prayers,

      Nancy

****

July 28, 2000

Last night we started to watch the video of the movie "Anna and the King". Dick went to bed part way through, but I decided to finish it. It had quite a sad goodbye at the end between Anna and the king, and then there was a very sad song during the credits. (Why did I watch the credits?) The song was something about, "Why can't I be with the man I love?" Thinking of how much I am going to miss the man I love brought forth a great deal of tears.

This morning, I told Dick about the end of the movie and that I am going to miss him terribly, and that started us both crying. I think it is important to let that grief out; it will come sooner or later - or sooner <u>and</u> later, but I think I should try to avoid crying in front of Dick as much as possible. He needs to reserve his energy for other things.

****

August 1, 2000

Jeremy came home on Friday and his girlfriend Amanda came with him. We had a great day Saturday. Dick had been miserable Friday morning, but had little pain on Saturday. He and Jeremy went out for breakfast while Amanda and I enjoyed fruit and conversation on the deck. We had other good conversations during the weekend also, including during the time we spent painting the wheelchair ramp. We had been told that we would need to sprinkle sand on the wet paint in order to make the surface less slippery for the wheelchair. It seemed silly to buy a large portion of sand for such a small job, so instead we went out to the street to gather sand left by the work crews when they had patched the asphalt on the road. We then sat in the "auxiliary driveway" (the part with the crushed stones) and sifted the sand through kitchen strainers to get all the big "impurities" out. We felt like a couple of kids playing in the sandbox, but our efforts paid off. The wheelchair ramp not only looks good; it also has just the right amount of traction!

On Saturday, Bobbie called from Camp to say that Zach was not feeling well - severe headache and some nausea. She had gone up for the weekend to help with checking in the new campers, and since she knows Zach, she was paying particularly close attention to him.

On Sunday, Ray and Jan arrived back here, having driven through a torrential downpour in Connecticut with a broken windshield wiper on the driver's side of the car. It was not just a broken wiper, but a completely malfunctioning mechanism. They found some string, and with Tim holding one end of the string from the right front seat, Jan holding the other end from the seat behind Ray, and the middle of the string tied to the wiper, (Tim pull right, Jan pull left; Tim pull right, Jan pull left. . .) they managed to keep the windshield sufficiently clear of rain to assure that they did not have an accident.

I was very glad that Ray and Jan were here to comfort me when Bobbie called to say that she was taking Zach to the emergency room in Bridgton, Maine because he was not getting any better. The emergency room doctor there decided to do a CAT scan and a lumbar puncture to check for meningitis. I was able to talk to him to explain that Zach's father was dying (and had recently had these same procedures that Zach was about to undergo.) Bobbie stayed with Zach for those procedures and to see him safely admitted to the hospital. The diagnosis was viral meningitis, but the doctor wanted to keep Zach in the hospital until today to make sure that nothing grew on the culture for bacterial meningitis. Bobbie stayed up in Maine until midday yesterday. I am so very grateful that she could be with Zach when I could not.

Today Zach is being discharged, but with continuing headaches, he is obviously in no shape to go back to camp (lifeguarding and counseling), so Ray and Jan have gone up to pick him up and bring him back here. What would I have done if they had not been here?

Chapter 26

August 3, 2000

Things change so quickly sometimes! We had that wonderful day last Saturday when Jeremy was here, but on Monday, Dick felt miserable again and was unable to urinate. Sandy came to put in a catheter, and felt that it should stay in, because if she removed it, he might have the same problem again. He thankfully did not object to that, but having the catheter in does mean more work in caring for him. It is a bit more complicated to take showers now, but he does love his showers, so I like to be able to help him with that - even though at the beginning of the week he was taking three showers a day.

Another difficult and sad thing that changed this week is that it is becoming more difficult for Dick to concentrate. He tries to do things on the computer - formerly his haven - but now he may forget where some file is in the computer, or he tries to reconfigure something and loses his concentration in the middle of the process.

It has not helped that the weather has not been pleasant lately. Dick loves his walks in the Breezy 500, but they have not been possible in the rain.

With all that is involved in caring for Dick as well as buying supplies he needs, trying to think of foods he might like and doing extra laundry, I don't know how I could manage without all the help I have. It is a rare meal that I have cooked lately; most of it has been provided by friends - freshly delivered or from the freezer - or it has been restaurant food: take-out or leftovers. Ray, Jan and Tim have been extremely helpful - not at all acting like guests. They pitch in to help without being asked, and they stay with Dick if I need to go out.

One day last week I was trying to find something that Dick might enjoy eating; not much appealed to him. The one thing that sounded positive to him was clam chowder or oyster stew, but I did not know where to buy it or how to make it. Just before he had mentioned this, a friend had called to ask if she might prepare some food for Dick. She wanted to know what he might like to eat, but I really wasn't able to offer any suggestions. All I told her was that he liked sweet and sour chicken, but he had just had some of that, and he had had his fill after only a half a serving. Since I had almost discouraged her from making anything, I was rather amazed that she arrived Saturday morning bearing a hearty kettle of seafood chowder! Since that is not a food that one normally thinks of bringing to a sick person (chicken soup, yes, but seafood chowder?) I was forced to conclude that God was paying attention to Dick's desires and lovingly supplying this one by the thoughtfulness of a friend.

This morning I saw Dick sitting in his wheelchair with his head in his hands, and I asked him if he was praying or crying or sleeping. "I'm just dying," he said.

****

August 8, 2000

Last week I finally reached the point of emotional exhaustion, but God is good. Plans had already been made for Mary Ellen, my Mom and Dad, and possibly Ray and I to go to Camp of the Woods for a couple of nights, so Jan started "shadowing" me on Wednesday so that she could learn what she would need to do in order to care for Dick while I was gone. Although it was very difficult for me to leave him, I felt that for both Dick's sake and mine, I needed a break from the twenty-four hour a day care. I felt very comfortable leaving him in Jan's care since she is a physician, but more importantly, she is loving and competent.

I left for my sister's house to meet the rest of the family mid-morning on the appointed day; Ray had gone out ahead of me. I cried for about the first half hour of the trip, and then decided that that was rather unproductive. I reasoned that the purpose of my going away was to get rest and refreshment, and this could not happen if I continued to cry. For the second half of the trip, I decided to have a chat with God. I realized that He had orchestrated the timing of this trip; He had clearly provided Jan, who could also keep an eye on Zach during his recovery; He had made Dick aware of my need to go and given him the love and grace to allow me to go; it was a good thing to be spending time with my parents; and on top of all that, Jesus had died for the guilt that I felt - reasonable or unwarranted. After thinking all that through, I arrived at Mary Ellen's house sober, but willing to make the most of the trip, which turned out to be quite enjoyable and refreshing.

One morning at a camp meeting, a man sang a song about how there will be no more tears or pain when we see Jesus. I do want that for Dick, though I don't want him to leave me. Now we can still talk things out, but there may come a time when even that will no longer be possible. His mobility will be less, and then, for both our sakes and for

Jeremy and Zachary, I hope he goes quickly. God has the day marked on His calendar, but He doesn't choose that we be privy to it.

Last Friday, when we were gone, Jan took Dick into his office because he seemed really anxious to go; he said something to Jan about only having a few days left. She brought Zach along to help Dick with whatever it was he wanted to do in his office, although Zach continued to have a headache. Jan said that Dick sat at his desk, going through piles of mail. He would pick up a publication - still in its plastic wrap - look at it for a moment, and then toss it in the trash, musing, "All this used to be so important to me."

Zach, meanwhile, lay on the floor of Dick's office in an attempt to quiet the pounding in his head. At one point, Dick apparently suddenly realized that Zach was there, not feeling well, and apologized for taking so long. "It's okay, Dad," Zach replied. "I'm okay. You take your time."

Jan says she saw in that exchange an older man and a younger man, very similar to each other, each wanting to put the other first. She noted that while Dick was no doubt proud of the computer chip that he had developed, how much more important to him were these "chips" - Zachary and Jeremy - into which he had invested so much more of his life.

Yesterday, Mary Ellen and Phil were here, and Dick talked with Phil about finances. Dick wanted to be sure that someone besides me understands the financial things, because when it gets beyond a simple checking account, I tend to get overwhelmed. After we all had spoken together and Dick was resting, the rest of the adults in the family stood around our pool table, and Mary Ellen asked what else they could do to help me. I told them that because of my inability to deal well with crises in the night, I did not want to ever spend another night alone with Dick. "You won't," she responded. I feel so blessed to have my family around. It is completely remarkable to me that we, who have been so far apart geographically for so many years, should all be together now at this most critical time in my life.

Yesterday I increased the amount of pain medication in Dick's patch. Last night he tossed and turned a great deal in bed - very unusual, since he is usually quite still when he sleeps. At about 3:30 AM he started talking about space and about his arm, something that made sense to him, but not at all to me. He started to become quite agitated, talking loudly and very crossly. He just wanted me to do what he wanted, but I could not understand what that was. I asked if he wanted pain medicine; he replied that he did, and he just wanted to get up. I have never been good with crises at night, and this was no exception. I started crying, borderline (?) hysterically, and went to wake Ray and Jan, but Jan was already halfway down the stairs. As soon as I started crying, it seemed to suddenly make Dick alert and aware, and he apologized, "I'm so sorry!" I was not able to stifle my hysteria as quickly, but did manage to get Dick's pills for him while Jan sat with him. She continued to stay with him while Ray listened to me cry and attempted to soothe my troubled spirit. Just having Ray and Jan here made such a difference for me in getting through that upsetting experience.

Even so, I had difficulty getting back to sleep after that whole incident because Dick was breathing quite loudly and slowly. I finally put ear plugs in my ears, assuming that I would awaken if I was needed. I did wake up when he needed pain medicine at 6:30. He still seemed anxious, though not as bad as earlier, so after I gave him some morphine, I removed the extra pain patch I had put on yesterday. The patches are supposed to last three days, but we have had to make adjustments from time to time.

For the rest of the day, Dick has been confused / cloudy. He still knows us all, but he seems to have some addition to reality in his thinking. For example, after Jan and Ray gave him his egg and toast for breakfast, he said, "Now can somebody do a simulation of how this is supposed to be done?" This afternoon after watching the TV show "Matlock" with Zach, Zach found him apparently pondering something. Slowly, with many pauses, he told Zach that he had been thinking: he couldn't remember why he had to prove by 11:00 tomorrow that the gun he owned was not the one used in the murder. Zach pointed out that he had fallen asleep during "Matlock", and maybe that was confusing him. He agreed, but said that it was a fun puzzle to figure out!

This morning as we were about to leave for our walk, he suggested that we pray. He prayed, "Lord, I think this is it. I know I'm confused. Thank you for Nancy." So sweet. So sad.

John, Susan and Elizabeth arrived here at about 6:00 PM. Everyone assisted with house clean-up and supper - very helpful. Dick mainly wanted to be with me. It is very difficult for John to see his brother like this.

I called Jeremy tonight. He and Liz plan to leave Virginia for home tonight. He was going to rent a van to bring with him all the equipment he will need to work out of home, but I had suggested yesterday that he not do that until he goes back to Virginia to work August 21-25. It should be more clear by then how Dick is doing - how long he is going to last.

When I talked to Jeremy tonight, I said that if the worst case occurred and his dad did not make it through the night, at least Jeremy could recall the great last weekend they had together. He responded that it would "suck" if he didn't make it back in time, and that I should tell Dad that he would be home in a half a day. I told Dick to hold on if he wanted until Jeremy comes and he said, "Definitely!"

Tonight after John left to go to his motel, Zach and I had a good talk. He decided, despite being headache free today, not to go back to camp. He would like to return to camp for the last weekend (August 19 and 20). We talked about the probability that it would be just the two of us living here in the fall and for the next school year. I told him that I will try to be a good mom, but I'm not a very good dad. He said he thinks that Dad did all the fathering he needed to do. He also told me that he has it all figured out what he will say when he comes upon a group of people crying about losing Dick. He'll say, "My father is not dead; he is singing and dancing in the presence of Almighty God!"

****

August 10, 2000

Dick awoke at about 4:00 yesterday morning, and he was a bit concerned. He said, "I have to talk to you. We need to talk privately." I assured him that everyone else in the house was in other rooms sleeping, so he continued, "I'm concerned about Mom's memory."

"Do you mean my mom?"

"Yes, and how it is affecting other people."

"Like my dad?"

"Yes, and other people."

I sensed he was concerned about his own memory loss, and I asked if I could comment.

"Certainly."

I told him that he was having some confusion and memory loss for a few reasons: the tumors, the medications, and maybe from his kidneys not working well and producing a chemical that could add to the problem. I assured him that it was okay for him to have memory loss, because he had taken care of all he needed to. I reminded him that everyone to whom he had spoken about finances had said that he had prepared very well for his family. I told him a little bit about my conversation with Zachary, and he seemed calmer and went back to sleep.

216

What a gift to be able to have conversations like this with my dear husband! I can't imagine going through this whole experience if Dick was in a hospital instead of at home with us. I am so very grateful for hospice and family who have made it possible for Dick to live his last days or weeks or however long he has at home.

Jeremy and Liz arrived at about 6:30 AM yesterday; they had really rushed to leave after my last phone conversation with Jeremy, and made the trip in record time. Dick awoke shortly after they arrived and really perked up - much more clear than the previous day. He remained quite animated for the remainder of the day, enjoying a half of a special Hoffman's / Heid's hot dog that John and Susan had brought from Syracuse.

John, Susan and Elizabeth went to Plimoth Plantation yesterday, but we had plenty of people around; Sandy came (I had told her a week or two ago that I wanted her to come more often than she had been coming - what a great support!) and Bob Ludwig visited to continue his discussions with Dick about planning the memorial service. Bob told us that he had recently given a sermon at a large church in the area and had used us as an example of people who were "transparent" during a time of trouble. I hadn't thought of it that way, but it is true. Dick is generally quite a private person, but he has been openly sharing his experience with so many people via email and the web page.

Today Dick was even brighter than yesterday, but he didn't eat anything until suppertime. The whole family was seated around the table on the deck, and I was sitting next to Dick, both of us facing away from the house, looking into the woods. I had put his pills (the Decadron and the one for nausea) on his plate, but just after he put them in his mouth, he spit them out, saying they were "too salty". I calmly explained why it was important that he take the pills, whereupon he picked them up off his plate and flung them across the table and off of the deck! It was a delightful show of chutzpah, greatly cheered by his brother-in-law, but I was not really sure of what he was saying. Was it just that the pills did not go down easily or tasted bad, or does he want to boycott pills now as a way of saying, "Enough! I'm ready to go"? I did not want him to miss the benefits of pain medication, so this evening we switched to liquid morphine, after which he requested "liquid water" as a chaser since the morphine did not taste good.

****

217

August 11, 2000

Dick awoke at 4:00 this morning, with an uncomfortable feeling that he had to urinate, even though he has a catheter. I was unable to irrigate his catheter, and although Jan was more successful, it was still apparently clogged, so one of the hospice nurses came to change it. Even after the change, he has had very little output.

He has continued to be quite uncomfortable all day, but we did attempt a family walk, which turned into quite an escapade. Jeremy, Zach and I and our dog Casper went out with Dick in "the Breeze". We had traveled about a half a mile when it started to sprinkle. Figuring that Zach was the fastest runner, we sent him back to get an umbrella. He returned with a huge umbrella and the car. We knew we would not be able to get Dick into the van, since he can no longer stand, so Zach took Casper in the car and left Jeremy and Dick and me with the umbrella. It was raining quite hard by the time we got home. It wasn't our best walk ever, but it was an adventure!

Dick's urine output continues to be very low, and Ray and Jan think that unless his urine output increases, it is unlikely that he will live more than a few days.

****

August 12, 2000, 12:05 AM
Email from me to friends (50 on list now)
Title: "God's love with skin".

I talked about the many ways I had experienced tangible expressions of God's love to me through the help of so many family members and friends in recent weeks as Dick's condition has changed. I told of the refreshment I received from going to Camp of the Woods with my family, and then I concluded the letter as follows:

Nonetheless, these past few days have not been easy, as Dick continues to grow weaker, have pain and experience confusion at times - more often than not some days. It is difficult to feel like a Ping-Pong ball being passed back and forth between the paddles of hope and despair. He seems to take 3 steps backward and then one step forward - or sometimes 2 steps forward or only 1/2 step sometimes. It is a difficult dance to follow.

I'm concerned for Jeremy, who had made his decision to stay home this next year, and had a job lined up working from home in Massachusetts for the Virginia architectural firm for which he worked this

218

summer. Now there is a possibility that Dick will not survive much beyond the summer, and Jeremy must decide again what to do. Both boys are being forced to deal with some pretty heavy stuff this summer, but they are responding with great maturity and tenderness towards both their parents.

Again, I can't thank you enough for your thoughts, prayers, and support - God's love in your skin.

Love,
Nancy

Rainbow:

August 2000 - January 2001

Chapter 27

August 12, 2000

Dick awoke once during the night needing pain medicine, but his bladder pain was much improved, and his urine was flowing bright orange, from a new medicine he is taking for bladder spasms. He awoke again at 6:30 AM concerned about Charlie (who is Charlie?) but agreed to go back to sleep and worry about it later.

When we all awoke after a decent length's sleep considerably later, Dick was quite bright and anxious to get going. Jeremy has been helping quite a bit with his dad's personal care since he came home, and today we decided to do Dick's sponge bath in bed. It was a rather jolly time; Dick wasn't clear that he had only one head - he thought he might have six or eight. Jeremy and I pointed out that there were eight heads in the house, and I asked if he knew who was here.

He said, "Nancy and Jeremy and me."

I asked him if he knew who was in the rest of the house, and he said, "Ray and Mary Ellen."

I corrected him, "No, not Mary Ellen, but Jan is here."

He tried again, "Phil's not here."

"No, Phil's not here." Just then we heard a loud sneeze from the kitchen.

"Ray's here!" he correctly concluded.

He wanted to get up and get dressed to go for a walk, and he even expressed interest in talking to his mother when I called her, but when he finally did get up, he was tired. Zach and I took a walk with him, but we turned around after going only about a quarter of our normal route because Dick was cold.

He continued to say a few funny and a few "off the wall" things today. Zach was with Dick when Jeremy came home from the store and inquired, "How are you doing, Dad?"

Dick turned to Zach: "Doesn't that kid know any other questions? He says 'How are you doing Dad?' every time he sees me!"

At one point after sleeping, he was a bit agitated. He told Ray that he had some important decisions to make. When I came in, he told me that he had decided that we didn't need to go through with the Bar Mitzvahs for the boys, "what with being Catholic and all." (?!)

A little later, when I returned to him after being out of the room, he made it clear that he was ready to go. "Nance, please help me die," he pleaded. After assuring him that I would do all I could to keep him comfortable, and giving my "permission" for him to go, I asked if he would like for us all to come in and pray with him. Without hesitation, he said "yes." Sometimes the whole bunch of us can be a little overwhelming for him. He's generally happy with just Jeremy, Zachary and me, but Ray, Jan, Tim and Elizabeth have been such a part of our household this summer, that I know he values their presence, too.

It must have been about 9:00. The living room was lit only by light spreading in from the kitchen and the street lamp outside. Dick lay on his side of the futon, the empty catheter bag hooked to the bed frame, a reminder of the failure of his body to complete the most basic of bodily functions. The bag has been empty all day. He ate nothing today, and drank only a little.

The boys knelt by the side of the futon and I sat on the end, while Ray, Jan, Tim and Liz finished out the circle. I prayed first – for an end to Dick's pain and for God to take him home soon. He prayed next – a clear prayer of thanks for his family and a desire to go now. In light of his confusion today, his clear prayer was especially precious. The boys prayed, too, and then Jan, and no doubt there were many silent prayers raised from that room as well. As we prayed, he put his hand of blessing on each of the boys and me.

After I prayed again – that we would be able to accept God's will if Dick wakes up again in the morning, improved, or still in pain – I started singing his favorite song: "Great is Thy Faithfulness". He joined in right away – in a little different key – and then several others joined the singing in *different* keys, and with somewhat varying words. Unfortunately, that Kline giggle kicked in for both Jeremy and me, but the others finished the song, followed by Dick's comment: "Well, He got the idea!"

We stayed in the room quietly for a while, and then filed out one at a time. Zach left last, knowing that this might be his last chance to say something to his father. "I love you, Dad," he whispered softly.

"I love you, too, Zach," answered Dick. Emotion filled his voice, but no more words were needed.

We reconvened briefly in the kitchen, where Ray commented, "There's no unfinished business here!" To be able to say good-bye with no words left unsaid, no regrets in our relationships - no "unfinished business" – is indeed a gift.

****

August 13, 2000 - Sunday

I woke up this morning frankly disappointed that God has not chosen to take Dick home yet. I know that none of us deserves any favors from God, but I also feel that Dick doesn't "deserve" to be in pain. It is so hard to remember that God's timing is perfect when His plan does not seem obvious to me.

I am reminded of the time between Jeremy's and Zachary's births. I had such a difficult time with Jeremy's birth that I didn't want to get pregnant again if the second experience was going to be a repeat of the first. Consequently, I went to the most conservative of the doctors in the group of obstetricians I knew, and asked him if he thought I would have the same problem (preeclampsia / hypertension in pregnancy) again for a second pregnancy. He told me that if I had underlying hypertension, the chances of the problems occurring again were quite high, but if I didn't, then the chances of it happening again were "practically nil". I proceeded to have liver function studies done (blood tests) and I decided to have my blood pressure checked regularly, praying that if I had underlying hypertension and was going to have problems with another pregnancy, that God would make that clear, so I wouldn't go through that again. The blood tests and blood pressure checks were fine, so in time I got pregnant again - and had trouble again. I was a little angry at God, as I recall, that He hadn't gotten my point! I didn't think about it again until Zachary was a couple of years old. One day I realized that if God had answered my prayer in the way I had wanted, I would not have this wonderful child!

We can't always see it while we are in the middle of difficult circumstances, but God's timing is best, and His ways are so much higher and better than ours.

Last night, after we prayed, Dick had pain medicine at 10:30 and then again at 12:30. At 1:00, Jeremy was still awake in the family room, and Zach was sleeping in the living room with us on a mattress on the floor. (We had recently agreed that the boys would take turns sleeping in the room with us in case I needed help during the night.) I had a nightmare. I dreamed that I got up, and when I came back to the living room, the futon on which Dick and I had been sleeping was folded up, and Dick was gone. Zach was in the bathroom, and I tried to knock on the door to get his attention, because I could hear Dick falling down the basement stairs. I was unable to knock, so I tried to scream for Jeremy,

223

but no sound came. I guess a sound finally did come out, because Dick woke me up and said, "What's wrong?"

"I just had a dream," I replied.

"That was easy!" was his relieved response.

Who is going to wake me up from my nightmares when Dick is gone? After the nightmare, Dick only awoke once; it was just a groan or some little noise that awakened me. I asked if he was in pain, but he said, "No." He didn't wake up again after that.

Early this afternoon, I realized that he was not going to wake up, at least not on his own. I felt it was time to turn and clean him, so with family help, I did that. He groaned when we first turned him, so I gave him more pain medicine, and then waited for that to work before the "big" turn. When four of us executed the big roll, he let out a wail / moan / groan that was heart wrenching, but short lived. He has seemed to be pain free otherwise; at least we hope so. There are some small moans, but Ray says he feels that if there is pain, Dick is perceiving it at a distance.

Dick's pulse is now unpalpable at the wrist and his heart rate has been quite rapid for a couple of hours. The boys and I turned and washed him again a little while ago, and now I have parked myself here with Dick, on the edge of the futon, to write and read; Jeremy is next to the futon working on the computer; and Zach is next to his dad eating ice cream and reading Calvin and Hobbes. We're listening to the Messiah, and I have this notion - still trying to plan God's timing - that Dick will go during the Hallelujah Chorus. It's a vigil we are keeping - a death watch, I guess - but we are so grateful that he does not seem to be in pain.

Well, the Hallelujah Chorus came and went. At the last strains, we all looked expectantly at Dick, expecting to see his final breath, but then the music stopped, and the next breath came. "Not God's timing," Jeremy said.

****

August 14, 2000
Email from me to friends
Title: "Graduation Day"
Dear Friends,

Today at about 12:35 am, Richard Burton Kline II graduated from the School of Humanity and immediately began his post graduate work in

Heaven. I expect that he was greeted with the words, "Well done, good and faithful servant."

I described the last two evenings of Dick's life in the letter and then continued.

The boys and I had a very strong sense of joy for him: he will never again experience pain or tears. We have cried our tears, and will no doubt cry many more as we miss this wonderful husband and father, but for now, the tears are dry. Richard Kline is with his Creator and Lord.

He will be cremated, and the Memorial Service will be held on Saturday morning, August 26 at 11:00 am at First Baptist Church in Foxboro. There will be calling / visiting hours at the church on Friday, August 25 from 6-9 pm. (The delay is because the church was not available the previous weekend, and Dick had wanted the service to be on a Saturday for ease of travel.)

So Graduation is over, but if you are available and want to join us in honoring the graduate, you are most welcome. Because many of you live at a distance or may not be available, please know that I will not interpret your absence as a lack of support! You have stood with us in thought and prayer for a long and sometimes difficult journey. Thank you from the bottom of my heart.

Love,
Nancy (for the Kline and Downing families)

****

How do people deal with death without the Hope of Heaven? If death were final, this day would have been the worst of my life, but in actuality, it was nowhere in the top ten list of "Nancy's Worst Days". There have been so many special gifts during these past months: some of the best times together ever for Jeremy and Dick; a solid sense of community support; being sheltered under a canopy of prayer; an opportunity to see the <u>exquisiteness</u> of God's timing (Ray and Jan here, the Camp of the Woods trip, Zach's meningitis, the whole thing being during school vacation for the boys and me); Dick's clarity for that final time of prayer; and even the fact that I was awake for his final breath.

May I remember these gifts and God's ever present Grace as I face the inevitable frustrations of life when I move back from "the valley of the shadow of death" to the road that is full of the distractions of this life. May I remember to turn my eyes daily, moment by moment, to Jesus.

THROUGH THE BARREN TREES

****

August 15, 2000
I got a little glimpse this morning of life's continuation after the relief and joy of Dick's graduation. Casper and I took a walk, following the route that we had been taking nearly daily with Dick in his wheelchair. It was a different route from the one I used to walk alone, because with Dick in "the Breeze", we had to find a route with less bumps. I considered this morning's walk a victory lap: Dick won the race and we took one more turn around the track. I cried with sadness that I would never walk that route with him again, and I cried for joy because he will never have to be in a wheelchair again. "Those who hope in the Lord will renew their strength. They will soar on wings like eagles; they will run and not grow weary; they will walk and not faint." (Isaiah 40:34) Dick will never be weak again.

Many people called, visited, and brought or sent flowers and food today. So many people are concerned. It could be overwhelming, but I try to remember that these folks are hurting, too, and since I am not at my most hurting moment, I need to minister to them.

One of the best calls today was from Rashid, Dick's boss in Arizona. He said Dick was not only a colleague but a friend as well. He spoke very highly of him and told me of some work that Dick had done before he died that would make it possible for the company to continue to develop the next phase of the "chip" for which Dick was the principal architect. This development might have been difficult without his recorded plans.

****

August 18, 2000
I received a most amazing letter today from our friend Dawn. Although Dawn had been very supportive by sending us numerous cards, we had not spoken much in recent months. The letter was dated August 16.

I am writing...to first communicate my joy and peace that Dick is busy praising God with the angels in Heaven...I love you and also hurt for your loss of him here...and I promise to continue to pray for you...

I wanted to write secondly about what happened on Sunday and Monday as I was praying for Dick...

A little history: I have been praying for Dick daily for months and months. For some reason, God's reason, Dick and your family danced across my mind at countless moments. Many times on my commute to work I would pass Washington Street [a main street near us] and this would be my trigger to pray. (Sometimes I would drive by your house praying. I think it was a small miracle your neighbors never reported me for stalking or "casing the joint" or that I did not set up a crash course with some innocent bystander.) The prayer times kept growing longer - sometimes I could not even concentrate on anything else. At one point I was afraid I was becoming obsessed (a social worker gone bad) but when I prayed about that, I received an increased passion to keep praying. At one point you mentioned how unbelievable it is that people pray for each other beyond their own lives, etc. I can't really say it had anything to do with me as to why I kept praying; I believe it was God's leading, not my own, and that for His purposes both for Dick, and what He wanted me to learn, kept me going.

On Monday morning / Sunday night at about 12:15 before bed I prayed that Dick would no longer be in pain and that the Lord would greet him home soon. I prayed this because I could no longer pray for anything else. When I would try, I kept getting a feeling that I was praying out of God's will. I could only pray for you and the boys and for Dick's comfort and arrival home in Heaven. I had prayed on and off since Saturday with the same general feeling, but it was very intense on Sunday night. About 12:40, I must have fallen asleep; it was about the time I set my alarm for Monday morning.

On Monday, I went through the day as usual. When I passed by Washington Street, I only prayed for you and the boys and Dick's mother and extended family. On the way home, I passed Washington Street again - this time with a flood of scriptures passing through my head. . . Then a song I have not heard in years about being still in God's presence came into mind; I sang it and then Great is thy Faithfulness - with all the verses - some I can't recall now. A few tears fell. I felt sort of shaken. Steve [Dawn's husband] got in my car... I told him what had happened. I told him I believed that Dick was in Heaven, although I felt a bit odd saying it, afraid that if he hadn't left for Heaven yet, I sounded like a nut. He was quiet as I went through exactly what happened. When we got home, my mom sent me on some quick errand, meanwhile telling Steve that Dick had passed... I actually had confirmation of the "graduation" of Dick at 9PM on Monday. I don't know when you updated the web site; I checked Tuesday. I found the coincidence of the hymn very wild, but very much like a God who tends to surprise us.

She continued on, promising to continue to pray for us. What a remarkable story!

Chapter 28

August 19, 2000

The past few days have been incredibly busy, with people calling and stopping to see me practically non-stop. Interestingly, my closest friends are the ones who have not called as much, giving me a little (much-needed!) space. They know that I will call if I need them.

Ray, Jan, Tim and Liz left Thursday morning for Arizona, where they plan to vacation as well as interview with the Indian Health Services for jobs there starting a year from now. They plan to return the night before the memorial service. It still amazes me how the timing for their visit here and their trips elsewhere in the U.S. coincided so beautifully with Dick's and my need for help. I really don't believe that was coincidence!

Thursday and Friday, when it was just Jeremy and Zachary and I here, we spent quite a bit of time making more arrangements for the memorial service. Although Dick had planned the bulk of the service and discussed that with Bob, there were still things we had to do. We decided that instead of buying flower arrangements for the church or ordering prayer cards, our "gifts" would be to put together photo displays and displays of Dick's work accomplishments and also to make a nice program for the service. We felt that a program would be more practical than a little card with a poem or a verse on it with his name. We reasoned that we could put a nice picture of Dick on the front, include the order of service and a letter to the attendees in the middle, and put the obituary on the back. That way, if people wanted to save it they could, but if they didn't, they could just treat it as a regular church bulletin and throw it away.

It really was a joy putting the displays and the program together. We looked through all our photo albums, enjoying the process of finding a combination of pictures: some heartwarming, some funny, and some just nice. We found a great picture for the front of the bulletin, and another one to prop up in front of the box with Dick's ashes. With the scanner that Dick bought and the new photo quality printer (that is now finally working well) Jeremy was able to enlarge some of the pictures that we chose, so we were able to make two really nice photo displays.

It has been interesting gathering things to highlight Dick's accomplishments. He has many patent awards and several photos of electronic chips that he designed. Because the kind of technical work he did was far beyond my comprehension, I called some of Dick's coworkers to try to get them to explain - in layman's terms - what he did. Because they are all so smart and technical, too, this was a challenge, but they were very helpful. They also had some very nice things to say about Dick, most notably how very bright he was. I also have received several notes from people who have worked with Dick, and many of them commented on Dick's character as well as his brilliance.

We haven't had the program printed yet; Jeremy is going to bring it to a printing place with which he has dealt in Charlottesville when he goes back there today. There are still things to be done, but we have another week before the memorial service. I am so very grateful for the time we have to do everything. I can't imagine what it would be like to have a loved one die suddenly, with no advance plans having been made for a service. Besides that, most people are buried rather than cremated, so one would not have the luxury of nearly two weeks for preparations before a funeral service was held. It seems odd even to me that I would call this a "luxury". Before Dick died, he talked about having the memorial service on a Saturday so that it would be easier for people who would be coming from a distance. I was a bit horrified, wondering what on earth I would do if he died at the beginning of a week: how could I wait that long for "closure" after his death? In reality, since our goodbyes to Dick occurred before he died, "closure" is not even an issue for me. He will never really be gone from my life, so I am grateful for this time to plan well his final celebration.

Another thing I had wondered about in years past was the issue of cremation versus burial. I have always felt that cremation made sense for a lot of reasons, but the most compelling one for me was my strong belief that our earthly bodies are not really us; they are just the houses that God gives us to use while we are here on earth. Though I believed this strongly, I did not know if I would feel differently if I lost someone close to me. In fact, the night Dick died, my convictions were solidified. When Dick breathed his last breath, I knew he was no longer in that body. Jeremy and Zach and I all had a strong sense that he was free, that he would never again feel pain, and that the body that was on the bed was just his house, and he had moved out. Because we knew that, we did not cry that night. If the nurse or the funeral director who came that night thought the absence of tears odd, they did not say so; they could not have been more supportive and kind.

Zachary left for camp yesterday to pick up his car, left there when he came home from the hospital in Maine, and Jeremy went back to

Virginia for his final week of work before returning for the memorial service. We were able to register him for the fall semester at UVA; there is really no reason now for him to not go back. Zach will be back tomorrow, so for a couple of days I am on my own - but hardly alone. I continue to have visitors, and there is plenty of work to do around here to keep me busy.

****

August 23, 2000

It is good to have this second week before the service. Zach came home on Sunday, and we have had a couple of days now with just the two of us - a little hint of what it will be like in the fall. I've been busy cleaning and preparing for next weekend and receiving calls and visitors but I also have had a little time to reflect. One thing I have been thinking about is how I would respond to a friend or acquaintance if he or she lost a loved one. People have been very thoughtful and caring, and I think this experience has enabled me to sort out what I have found most helpful, and consequently how I think I might express my condolences.

1 - I would send a card - soon. I'd send a note if I didn't have a card. We have received over 120 cards. Sometimes, I don't have a chance to read them until a day after they come, but I can read them when I have time. I can sit and think about each one. A card, unlike a phone call, doesn't go away when another card or phone call comes. If I knew the person who died, I would write on the card some memory about that person or note why that person was special. I've gotten some wonderful notes about Dick.

2 - If I saw the person who lost the loved one, I would say, "I'm so sorry" if the person was just an acquaintance. The grapevine is big in Walpole, and I daily see someone who knows about Dick's dying, and these people have been kind.

3 - If I knew the person a bit better, and I saw them and I knew they didn't have trouble with touch, I would give a hug. I've gotten hugs from people who wouldn't normally be huggers, and that has been good.

4 - If it was a close friend who had lost someone close, I would make a quick call and not mind being put off or cut off and would not expect a call back, but I would try to make myself available. I might not even call right away, but first send a note or email - or two. This is what my close friends have done.

231

5 - Would I send flowers? I don't know. I really like flowers, and I am grateful for each bouquet I have received, but there is not much room left to put them. Maybe I'd bring over a single rose, or maybe send flowers in a month or two - maybe on the deceased person's birthday, if I knew it. Fruit is also a nice idea.

6 - If I made some food, I'd put my name on the dish if I expected it to be returned. I have a bunch of dishes for whom I don't know the owner.

7 - If I bought a plant, I'd add a card with my name. I have a lovely plant - from ? I'd consider giving plants that could be planted outside. Most of mine can be.

8 - If I brought something, and I didn't know the recipient well, I might just put it in a bag with a note and put it inside the door without ringing the bell. One person did this: nice.

9 - I'd start a list of gifts when the first one arrived so I wouldn't forget who gave them. (Oops! That was one for me, not what I would do for someone else!)

10 - I might also give a meal gift certificate for a local restaurant, to be used whenever the bereaved person wanted. Someone did that for us: nice.

****

August 24, 2000

Bob called earlier today to see how I was doing, and Barb called this evening. I haven't cried much since Dick died, but I told Barb that I became a little sad walking today, thinking that Dick was my best friend and soul mate and that I was going to miss that special relationship. I told her that the feeling passed quickly as I realized how blessed I was to have had him as my husband for twenty four years - a marriage of a quality that some people never experience. When I was talking to Barb, though, I got really sad and teary. She was talking about the importance of experiencing grief, not putting it off or stifling it. I don't feel as though I have been trying to not feel grief, but I had cried only once in the ten days since Dick died. While I was talking to Barb and after, while looking at pictures of Dick, I saw the pictures differently than I had seen them when I was picking them out with the boys. Then, it was choosing a good variety of pictures. This evening it was as if I looked at the pictures and in some of them I saw him, not just a picture. That made me sad, realizing that he is really gone. I cried then and a little on the way to the

232

airport to pick up Jeremy and Amanda, and again when I saw Jeremy. Dear, <u>dear</u> boys - both of them. What a blessing!

****

August 27, 2000

The calling hours and memorial service were wonderful - a real tribute to Dick and I believe they were honoring to God as well. The programs that Jeremy had printed in Virginia came out beautifully; the paper and picture quality is so good that I believe one could frame the picture if he wanted. Jeremy, Zach, Amanda and I folded all 350 of them on Thursday night, and on Friday the boys and I set up the church for the calling hours while Amanda stayed back at the house and cut up fruit for after the service. I'm glad that we allowed three hours for visitors, because there was a steady stream of people the whole time, and we heard that the line even extended out the door at times. Having the displays gave people something to look at while they were waiting in line. The boys were great as they greeted people whom they had never met, as well as many of their friends. It was really gratifying to see the number of young folks who had the courage to come; I know it must not have been easy for them. One of Jeremy's friends took a bus across the country from Washington state to express his condolences. At Dick's request, the Messiah played continuously during the calling hours.

Yesterday, the day of the service, was indeed a memorable day. The boys, who had shaved their heads the night Dick died, shaved them again on Friday, in an act of respect. As a further demonstration of utmost respect, they chose to both dress all in black: black tuxedos, black shirts and black ties. Although they looked extremely handsome and respectful, I did have the feeling standing between them that I was being protected by a couple of Mafia bodyguards! I also had a sense, as I stood in the front row of the church between them with Dick's ashes and pictures of him in front of me, that somehow I was in the wrong picture; this should not be me, the central living person at a memorial service for the man I loved.

Nonetheless, the service itself was the celebration we had hoped it would be. It was beautiful, uplifting, sad, hopeful, elegant and simple from the lovely prelude music (including two songs from our wedding) to the triumphant strains of the "Hallelujah Chorus" for the recessional. Bob gave me a copy of his notes, which aren't exactly what he said, but they capture the essence of his messages. After we sang "Great is Thy

Faithfulness", and Ray read a few Scriptures, Bob spoke about who Dick was:

I learned of Dick's death while I was in Florida attending a conference. Although I had seen him just 5 days earlier and knew the end was coming, I was still devastated when I heard the news. That evening I withdrew from my conference for several hours and sat by the hotel pool just to reflect - reflect on Dick's life and reflect on life in general.

The next day I boarded a plane to head home. On the trip home I sat by myself and began to ask questions like: "What was the essence of Dick Kline's life? What made him tick? What motivated him? What shaped Dick? What made him become the man we all knew?"

I've known Dick for about 27 years. Over the last 10 days I have reflected back on times when Dick helped me in times of need. I thought of many great times shared together in the house church in Cambridge 25 years ago, and many annual reunions of the house church at Dick and Nancy's home here in Walpole over the last 19 years. I re-read the many messages and emails on the Kline website. I listened to The Messiah, which Dick listened to again and again during his last weeks and months. And I kept asking the questions, "What made Dick Kline tick? What was the essence of his life?"

After days of mulling over those questions, two phrases emerged from my thinking that I believe describe Dick:

1. Dick was a man who lived for others, and

2. Dick had an eternal perspective.

Bob went on to expand on both those things, citing examples of how Dick had helped other people and noting that his greatest concern as he was dying was not for himself - for his pain or what he would miss on this earth by dying - but rather that he was having to leave me alone and that he felt the boys had had to grow up faster than they should have.

He spoke about Dick's eternal perspective - that he had unshakable confidence that even if he were not cured of cancer, he would be okay. The persistent direction for his life was to glorify God, and he knew that his ultimate prognosis was eternal life.

We sang the three worship songs that Dick had picked out: "Knowing You", "Shout to the Lord", and "Awesome God" (complete with guitars, piano and drums) and then our good friend Paul spoke about Dick and how through their friendship and how Dick lived, he had taught Paul how to live. He told about a time that Dick had given him a hug that was not one of those "guy" hugs, but a healing hug, that shared Christ's love. He spoke of Dick's deep, abiding love for God, and noted that his faith was not "death denying" but rather "life affirming".

After Paul spoke, there was about a half an hour when different people got up to share their remembrances of Dick. There were quite a number of people who spoke: people from church, people who had been in Bible studies with us, family, and Dick's manager at Motorola - Rashid. The time of sharing gave wonderful glimpses into different aspects of Dick's life.

Bob's closing charge was particularly memorable. After some comments about Dick, Bob spoke first to his mother, then to the boys and me, and then to the whole congregation.

We've heard a lot about Dick Kline this morning - how he lived and how he died. So what should we learn from Dick's life?

I go back to one of the scriptures read for us earlier in the service: "I have fought the good fight, I have finished the race, I have kept the faith."

"I have fought the good fight." Dick certainly fought the good fight. The last 2 ½ years were one long fight. But he fought it and he fought it well.

"I have finished the race." Dick's race here on this earth is indeed finished. One of the awesome aspects of a memorial services like this is that we are able to see the end of someone's race and see if they finished well or not so well. Dick finished well.

"I have kept the faith." Dick's faith in Christ not only endured until the end, it sustained him, and it nourished him until the end.

I'd like to speak first to Mrs. Kline. Mrs. Kline, I can't imagine what it's like to lose a child that you have borne. But I know that God cares, and that His grace can uphold you. I wish God's blessing upon you as you deal with the loss of your son.

Jeremy and Zach, your Dad loved you very much. He was proud of the men you have become. My challenge to you is not to imitate his vocation or his hobbies or his interests. You need to become the men God has created you to become. But I do challenge you to imitate your Dad's character, and I challenge you to adopt his eternal perspective.

Nancy, Barb and I have known you since you were a college student struggling with your faith. And in the past 2½ years, you have demonstrated grace under pressure. You have showed us faith in the tough times.

Nancy, Dick was madly in love with you, but you know that; I don't need to tell you that. My challenge to you is to give yourself space to feel. You have put one foot in front of another, and you have done it admirably. But now allow your feelings to rise to the surface. Remember that through it all, you can trust God. God did not forsake you during the last 2½ years; He won't forsake you now.

And now, a challenge to all of us. Dick's finish is clearly saying something to us. I think it's saying, "Think about how you want to finish the race. Think about what you want people to say at your celebration service. Think about how you want to fight the last fight. Then figure out what you have to do now to get there. Then live your life today in a way that leads toward that end."

I am reminded of a poem by William Cullen Bryant called "Thanatopsis." It's a poem about death, and after discussing death throughout most of the poem, Bryant ends with a challenge to us who are living.

> *"So live, that when thy summons comes to join*
> *The innumerable caravan, that moves*
> *To that mysterious realm, where each shall take*
> *His chamber in the silent halls of death,*
> *Thou go not, like the quarry-slave at night,*
> *Scourged to his dungeon, but sustained and soothed*
> *By an unfaltering trust, approach thy grave,*
> *Like one who wraps the drapery of his couch*
> *About him, and lies down to pleasant dreams."*

I'd like to paraphrase the poem just a bit, but keep the same thrust.

So live... that when your summons comes to join the innumerable caravan that moves to that mysterious realm, you go having loved your family and friends. So live... that when your summons comes, you go with the knowledge that you have lived life to the full and become the person God created you to be. So live... that when your summons comes, you know that you have made a difference in other people's lives. So live... that when your summons comes, you go with a firm and unfaltering confidence in God your Maker.

So live... so live... SO LIVE!

Amen.

Chapter 29

September 4, 2000
Email from me to friends
Title: "Thank you"

Thank you for all your thoughts and prayers and cards in the past weeks. As those of you who were able to attend Dick's Memorial Service witnessed, it was, I believe, a real tribute to him and was glorifying to God as well. I think the words that were shared and the sense of celebration of his life that was felt will remain with me for a long time.

Tomorrow I officially go back to work. (I say officially, because I already went in once last week to open up my office and hook up my computer.) I think it is a good thing to be going back; the people at work are very supportive. Last week was kind of a transition week for me. My brother's family and Jeremy left on Sunday (the day after the service), and that was quite difficult. However, Liz, my niece, was here until I brought her back to BU on Saturday, so she, Zach and I had some good times together.

Perhaps the most memorable was last Sunday night (8/27). Dick and I had received a bottle of sparkling cider in a gift basket several months ago, and had been saving it for some sort of celebration - the end of radiation? family vacation? a day of feeling really good? Anyway, that celebration never came, so we still had the cider on Sunday night when there was ABSOLUTELY NOTHING to celebrate. So, for that very reason, we opened it, drinking it from our very best fine crystal wine glasses - while speaking in proper English accents, no less. It actually was fun!

I just had the sense that that is precisely the kind of choice I will need to continue to make on a regular basis. There is no doubt at all that I do and will miss Dick terribly; he was my very best friend. However, for whatever reason, God has chosen to give him the ultimate reward now, and it is His plan for me and the boys to continue on with life on this earth. I have no doubt that He did not make a mistake in that; He loves us and has special plans for us until He chooses to take us home also.

For now, Jeremy is back at school working hard and loving me from afar. Zach is loving me from nearby and preparing to start school on Wednesday. We have periodic short discussions on how this year *together can proceed as smoothly as possible. (So far, very good.) I've started my book about this whole cancer / faith / pain / joy / love experience, and though it may never be published, I think it will be good for me to review it and record it for Dick's descendants. (Tentative title: Grace in the Storm)*

I don't suppose I will keep sending these updates; Dick doesn't need our prayers any more, though I'd be grateful if you would continue to pray for me, the boys and Dick's family as you think of us from time to time. We have so very much appreciated your taking this journey with us.

Love and thanks,
Nancy

****

September 4, 2000
Ray sent me an email, and forwarded for me an email that he had received from his friend Michael Blanchard. What a lovely sentiment!

Mercy beyond words is my prayer for Nancy and her family and a whisper to her heart, like a breeze from the far country perhaps, a blown kiss from one "good and faithful servant" to another, a telegram printed on the soul maybe that reads..."arrived safe and sound stop it's more beautiful than i could have imagined stop all was, is, and will be, well...so wonderfully WELL start."

****

October 23, 2000
Jeremy flew in from Virginia last night, and today he, Zach and I went up to New Hampshire to scatter Dick's ashes. Dick always loved the mountains of New Hampshire, and he loved Camp Berea, so we chose the last mountain that he had climbed, Bear Mountain, just across from the Berea entrance and overlooking Newfound Lake, to leave the remains of his earthly home. It was a beautiful warm, sunny autumn day, and while the leaves did not have the brilliance of the early fall oranges and yellows, they glowed with bronze and golden hues. It was, as we had expected it would be, a good day, including times of sadness, gratitude and laughter. We met no one on the way up or on the way down the mountain. Two people came by after we had prayed and were in the middle of scattering the ashes, but they kindly did not stop, even though we were at the prime scenic overlook at the top of the mountain.

Months ago, when we had asked the funeral director what to do with the box that held Dick's ashes after we had scattered the ashes, he had suggested that we break up the box and leave it on the mountain, but we were unsuccessful in that venture, so we decided to adopt his second suggestion: burn it. As we quietly watched the box burn, Jeremy noted that fire is "contemplative" and Zach mentioned the burning bush, when God spoke to Moses. What an amazing way for God to show himself - in a fire that did not consume the bush, and was warm and beautiful, but could not be touched.

****

October 24, 2000

Zachary has written one of his essays for college entrance. Whether or not it gets him into college, this one was a real gift to me.

I consider myself to be very blessed. It's cloudy right now, but when my family and I sprinkled my father's ashes in New Hampshire yesterday the weather was gorgeous.

My father was a wonderful man. Some people, when they hear "You're just like your father" thrown at them, consider it a criticism. I consider it to be the highest praise. My father was humble, loving, intelligent, and possessed a wonderfully understated sense of humor. He graduated Summa Cum Laude from Syracuse University, second in his class, earned his master's degree at MIT, and led a Bible study every Tuesday night in the prison near our home. He holds seven patents in electronics and built the treehouse in our back yard. He died of cancer at 12:30AM on August 14, and currently resides in the presence of God Almighty.

I spend this time talking about my father in an essay about my goals and who I am because to me these subjects are critically intertwined. I do not wish to be my father, because I am a unique individual, but I aspire to someday be a man of his character. I consider myself privileged to have known this man for seventeen and a half years, and blessed to have had him as my father.

Who am I? I am Richard Kline's son and a child of God. What are my achievements? I was the recipient of Walpole High School's "Outstanding Freshman" and "Outstanding Junior" awards, I placed fifth in the Division II state wrestling tournament last year, and a little boy named Gabe says I'm good at piggyback rides. What is my goal? I

239

strive to live such an outstanding life that when I meet my Maker face to face He will say, "Well done, my good and faithful servant."

****

November 4, 2000
Zachary wrote another essay - this one for University of Maryland. It is a wonderful reflection of his writing ability, his faith and his love for his dad. If the University of Maryland does not accept Zach, I think it will be their loss!
My father is not dead.
Five months ago, the doctors told him he would die. My parents broke the news to me that night at supper, in air full of the scent of citronella candles and the sound of birdsong. You often hear it said about moments like these that "time stood still," or that "at that moment, time stopped". Those sayings are completely false. You try to stop, and time drags you along with it just the same. The clock in the dining room continues to tick away and strike regularly on the hour, days retain their habitual twenty-four hour cycle, the phone continues to ring and the mail to come every day at 11:00, and the rest of the planet rudely refuses to stop going on with everyday life despite your shocking news. Against my wishes, my life continued to slip away as well. I was in the middle of my final exams, and they had to be completed whether I liked it or not. Surprisingly, my finals went well, and the flurry of school's end parties and beach trips came and went also. After the initial shock of the news had passed, I embraced denial. It suddenly seemed to me that my dad and I had all the time in the world. I knew that he probably would not be here to see me graduate, but like his death, graduation seemed to be an event that would never come. I was a seventeen year old boy whose summer vacation had just begun, and everything I touched was immortal.
I went away to camp for a few weeks, then contracted viral meningitis and was hospitalized. Through that illness, God sent me a message. I realized that my body is not immortal, and neither was my father's. My illness forced me to return home just as he took a turn for the worse.
Over the next weeks I watched as my father's body slowly shut down. He was on high doses of morphine to deal with the pain, but the medicine didn't always stop his headaches. He lost the strength to stand, even with something to lean on, and then he stopped eating. At

times he became confused. He wasn't forgetful, but would make connections between unrelated things, like thinking TV characters were visitors. Two weeks after I returned home, he slipped into a coma.

My family has always been very close-knit and has always had a strong faith in God. My experiences in life have not destroyed the beliefs I was taught as a child, but have rather refined and strengthened them, and given them a more personal meaning to me. Throughout my father's illness, the rest of my family and I remained confident of the fact that God would always be with us and that no matter what we endured on Earth, we would all see each other again someday in Heaven. I still believe this with all my heart.

The next night, I was awakened about half past midnight by my brother. The room was dim, but enough light filtered in from the street that I could see him clearly. The house was quiet except for the ticking of the hall clock. As he leaned in through the doorway, I could see my father in his face.

"What?" I asked, though I already knew the answer.

"He's gone," my brother said softly. He did not say it tearfully, but rather quietly, as one who is revealing proof of long held suspicions does when he is not sure how the listener will react.

"Good," I said, peeling back my covers and standing up. We did not shed any tears that night. It was not a time of sorrow but of rejoicing. We had seen my father fading in pain, and had had the chance to say goodbye. He had been ready to go, and had said so. His pain had ended, and now he had been received into the place where tears and sorrow are no more. He was in the presence of Almighty God.

I said before that my father is not dead. He is not. Though his body has been destroyed and spread to the wind, he lives on. Without question I miss him, and I am at times sorrowful, but I comfort myself with the fact that I will see him again someday, and I like to think that perhaps he sees me now. I strive to live a life that will make him proud, and to use to the fullest the abilities that I have been given.

****

December, 2000
Christmas letter to friends
Dear Friends,

"My soul glorifies the Lord, and my spirit rejoices in God my Savior, for he has been mindful of the humble state of His servant. . . The Mighty

241

One has done great things for me – Holy is His name." It's often referred to as "Mary's song" – uttered when she found out she would be the mother of Jesus, our Savior, but I feel that I, too, can sing the same song this Christmas. Throughout Dick's illness, and since his death in August, I have been very aware of God's love for our whole family. In the midst of sadness, we have been able to rejoice, and after many times of frustration, we were able to recognize God's grace, and indeed recognize Him as the Mighty One. Holy is His name.

This fall has been a time of adjustment. Jeremy went back to school, though he had been prepared to take a year off to be with Dick. It took a little time to get back in the swing of things, but he's once again totally immersed in architecture. He received intermediate honors for his first 2 years of studies, and when asked by his cousin during Thanksgiving dinner what he would like to do if he could have any job in the world, he said he'd like to be an architect. How nice that he really enjoys what he is doing!

Zachary started the fall in a less hectic fashion than usual, since he chose not to play soccer this year. He was able to get a good start academically, and he took up judo, something Dick also enjoyed in high school. It was a good way to stay in shape in preparation for wrestling season, which is now underway. He was chosen as co-captain (reportedly unanimously) by his peers at the end of last season. He has nearly completed his college applications, focusing mainly on U Maryland, Virginia Tech and Lehigh, intending to study mechanical engineering.

I was happy to return to the very supportive community of my school, where this year has been much less busy than recent years. Paperwork at home, though, has seemed endless, leaving me little time to work on the book that I began writing just after Dick died. Consequently, I requested, and have been granted, a leave of absence extending from the school Christmas vacation until after February vacation to continue writing <u>Through the Barren Trees</u>, the story of our family's journey with cancer and faith. The book will be an expansion of the material in Dick's web page. Whether or not a publisher wants it, I think it will be worth my time to write it, perhaps having it self-published. I'm very much looking forward to this experience.

Christmas will surely be different for us this year; we do and will sorely miss Dick, but I am so grateful for the boys and so many wonderful family members and friends. We also rejoice that Dick isn't just listening to pretty Christmas music on CD's and driving around

242

looking at decorated homes this year; he's making music and celebrating with the One for Whom Christmas celebrations first began — Jesus Christ, the King of Kings!

May you know Joy and Peace in a special way this Christmas season and in the year to come.

****

January, 2001

This is not the end of my story. I miss Dick dreadfully at times, and sometimes I wonder how I will manage when Zach leaves for college in the fall. Despite my fears and sorrows, however, I have an absolutely unshakable confidence that the God who loved my dear husband loves me, too, and will never leave me. I cling to the many promises given in His Word, such as this one from Jeremiah 29:11, "'For I know the plans I have for you,' declares the Lord, 'plans to prosper you and not to harm you, plans to give you hope and a future.'" He does not promise a future without pain or problems, but I know from my experience through one of life's storms that His compassions never fail and His faithfulness is indeed great.

Printed in the United States
3552